Smart Eating

BOOKS BY COVERT BAILEY

Fit or Fat?
The Fit-or-Fat Target Diet
The New Fit or Fat
Smart Exercise

BOOKS BY COVERT BAILEY
AND LEA BISHOP

Fit-or-Fat Target Recipes
The Fit-or-Fat Woman

BOOKS BY COVERT BAILEY
AND RONDA GATES

Smart Eating

Smart Eating

Choosing Wisely, Living Lean

Covert Bailey
and Ronda Gates

HOUGHTON MIFFLIN COMPANY
Boston • New York

For information about permission to reproduce selections
from this book, write to Permissions, Houghton Mifflin Company,
215 Park Avenue, New York, NY 10003

For information about this and other Houghton Mifflin
trade and reference books and multimedia products, visit
The Bookstore at Houghton Mifflin on the World Wide
Web at http://www.hmco.com./trade.

Library of Congress Cataloging-in-Publication Data
Bailey, Covert.
Smart eating : choosing wisely, living lean / by
Covert Bailey and Ronda Gates.
p.   cm.
Includes index.
ISBN 0-395-75283-3
1. Weight loss.   I. Gates, Ronda.   II. Title.
RM222.2.B344   1996   95-37876
613.2 — dc20   CIP

Printed in the United States of America

QUM   10 9 8 7 6 5 4 3 2

ACKNOWLEDGMENTS

Every creative effort has a powerful behind-the-scenes support team. This book is dedicated to ours: Dave Fabik, Tami Jewell, Beth Morris, Cindy Stanley, and Marni Timm Wegener.

Contents

PART ONE

Covert's Target Rules

1

Good Foods, Bad Foods

CHOCOLATE CAKE AND TWINKIES may be junk food to you, but if you were stranded on a desert island they could mean the difference between life and death for at least a few days. Practically every "junk food" has some redeeming quality. You may scorn sugar, but it's THE FASTEST WAY to reenergize a worn-out hiker or a marathoner after a race. The fact that *you* don't need the extra calories does not make them "bad."

Foods that are highly touted for being "nutritious" often contain fewer nutrients than some fairly decent foods that we tend to sneer at. A fast-food hamburger, for instance, has far more nutrients than Mother Nature's fresh-picked apple. Fruit juices are nothing more than a smattering of vitamins in a solution of sugar and water.

Even foods that contain the highest concentrations of vitamins, minerals, and protein, such as liver and eggs, are not perfect — along with their goodness they often have some drawback, such as too much fat or cholesterol. Yet we wouldn't call them "junk" foods.

So let's get something straight:

FOODS ARE NOT GOOD OR BAD —
FOODS ARE GOOD AND BAD.

Every food contains some good stuff and some bad stuff. We need to find a way to label foods so that we can easily choose the ones that have more good stuff than bad.

A simple food diagram consisting of two pie-shaped wedges pointed at each other is a good way to illustrate this idea. The top wedge shows how much good stuff, or nutrition, is in the food, and the bottom one represents the bad stuff, or "empty" calories. Lemon Jell-O would look like this:

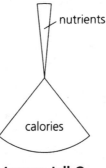

Lemon Jell-O

The skinny slice at the top represents the meager amount of vitamins and protein; the bottom wedge is fatter because Jell-O is mostly empty calories.

Liver would look like this:

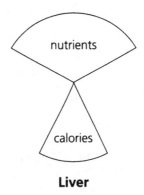

Liver

The top wedge is fat because liver is bursting with vitamins, minerals, and protein, but the medium-sized slice on the bottom shows that it is also high in cholesterol and fat.

Wouldn't it be neat if people had to wear such labels? Then we could look at our politicians and see at a glance whether their sugar-coated promises were balanced by good intentions.

Let's look at that apple again.

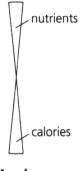

Apple

We all know that eating even twenty apples a day won't make us fat, so the pie at the bottom representing empty calories is very narrow. But the sliver on the top shocks people — apples contain very small amounts of vitamins.

How about a nice thick steak?

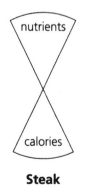

Steak

Terrible choice, you say, loaded with fat, bound to give you a heart attack. Yet beef contains one of the highest-quality proteins you can eat. The top wedge tells us that it has lots of vitamins, minerals, and protein, along with the grease shown by the wedge at the bottom.

These diagrams, neat as they are, are far from perfect. The upper wedge for a carrot may not be very large, but carrots contain so much vitamin A that one could supply all the vitamin A you need for a day.

Let's take another look at Jell-O. The wedge on the bottom is pretty big, but it doesn't tell us whether the calories come from sugar or fat. If I were a marathon runner I wouldn't think twice about eating extra sugar calories (if you want to know why, see pages 54–60 in *Smart Exercise*), but I would avoid extra fat calories. I'm sure you know that in Jell-O the calories are sugar, but what if it were an unfamiliar food?

The diagrams compare good stuff to bad stuff, but they leave us wondering which vitamins are represented in the top and where the empty calories in the bottom come from. To find out what each food contains, nutritionists look in thick books with endless boring tables of foods. Luckily there's a simpler way to get the same practical information.

Instead of listing all of the vitamins, minerals, and proteins in tables, foods can be arranged by groups based on their dominant nutrients:

Food Group	Dominant Nutrients
Meats	Protein, iron, niacin
Milks	Calcium, riboflavin, protein
Breads and cereals	B vitamins
Fruits and vegetables	Vitamin C and/or A

You should memorize the nutrients of each group so that if I say a food is predominantly a milk, you will know that it has calcium, protein, and riboflavin. Beans, even though they were "born" a vegetable, belong to the meat group because their dominant nutrients are protein, iron, and niacin.

Jell-O gives you almost none of the vitamins or protein associated with the food groups. It also has no fat; all of its calories come from sugar. We're urged to eat less fat, and some "nutritionists" even give clients lists of foods based solely on their fat content. Jell-O would look great on such a list, but it isn't great. Steak, on the other hand, would be a no-no because of its fat content, even though, as the earlier pie diagram showed, it has a substantial amount of nutrients.

Too many people trying to avoid fat overlook the necessity of getting nutrition from their food. Beef is both good *and* bad; Jell-O is *neither* good nor bad. What to do? Is there an easy way to look at foods and tell which ones have too much fat or sugar *and* make sure we get ALL the vitamins, minerals, and protein we need? You bet there is! Read on.

2

The Target Principles

I LIKE TO COMPARE smart eating to archery. To illustrate my approach I've created a Smart Eating Food Target with foods arranged according to their fat content. Most of the time we aim to eat the nutritious foods found in the bull's-eye, but occasionally we shoot a stray arrow into some high-fat ice cream or potato chips. As with archery, most of us expect to be off center once in a while. In fact, we get quite impatient with those "straight arrows" who can't enjoy eating or let us enjoy eating because they think every food selection must be perfect. Knowing that low-fat eating is good, they buy, cook, and eat nonfat everything.

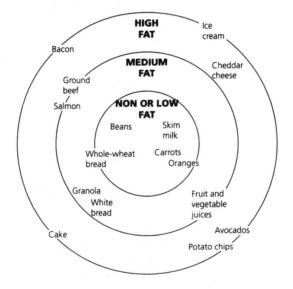

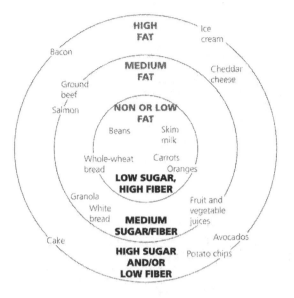

I eat nonfat selections from the bull's-eye when practical, but I include fattier foods in my diet when their taste and nutritional value justify it. Even that occasional wild arrow at a high-fat cheese or meat on the Target's outer edge can be justified if the rest of my day is balanced with low fat.

The neat thing about the Smart Eating Food Target is that we can also place foods according to their sugar and fiber content. Most foods that are high in fiber are also low in sugar, but as these foods are refined, their fiber content goes down and their sugar content goes up. Thus, whole-wheat products go in the bull's-eye, while refined white-flour products with added sugar are placed in the outer circles. Similarly, fruits and vegetables are bull's-eye foods, but their juices are not. Despite the claims of juicing advocates, as vegetables and fruits are squeezed or juiced, they lose their fiber, and the sugars are more concentrated. Orange juice contains vitamin C, of course, but it contains almost as much sugar as a soft drink. People who drink orange juice in the morning because they think their bodies are craving vitamin C are kidding themselves. Typically, blood sugar is low in the morning, and their bodies crave sugar! Better to have one orange with its high fiber and moderately

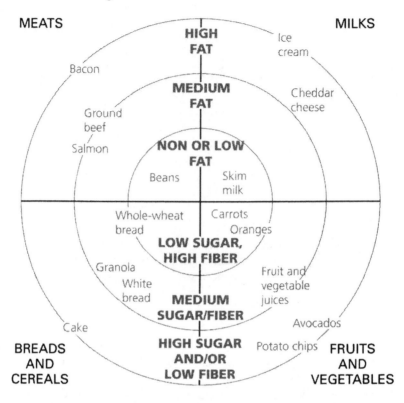

MEATS   MILKS

HIGH FAT
Ice cream

Bacon

MEDIUM FAT
Cheddar cheese

Ground beef

Salmon

NON OR LOW FAT

Beans   Skim milk

Whole-wheat bread   Carrots   Oranges

LOW SUGAR, HIGH FIBER

Granola

White bread   MEDIUM SUGAR/FIBER   Fruit and vegetable juices

Cake   Avocados

BREADS AND CEREALS   HIGH SUGAR AND/OR LOW FIBER   Potato chips   FRUITS AND VEGETABLES

low sugar than the concentrated sugar of four oranges squeezed into a glass.

By aiming for the center of my Target, you are changing three things about the food you eat: it's lower in fat, lower in sugar, and higher in fiber. However, an important nutritional concern is still missing. It's that age-old dictum our grandmothers espoused — *Eat a balanced diet.* Long before science proved it, grandma's common sense told her we need to eat a variety of foods to get all our vitamins and minerals and complete proteins. So I've added another wrinkle to the Target; I've divided it into quadrants to represent the four groups of food, and voilà! I've targeted the four basic food groups!

I like the Target concept because it illustrates, in one picture, the four important rules *all* nutritionists try to enforce. Notice that I said ALL nutritionists! People get so confused about the claims and counterclaims of different "experts" that they ignore the four rules the experts *don't* argue about. If you attended a nutrition conference in Guatemala or Russia or France, you would hear agreement on the four rules. No matter who you are — famous mountaineer or ordinary working stiff — *everyone* should live by the Target's four basic principles, and these will never change.

Eat a diet that is:

1. Low in fat
2. Low in sugar
3. High in fiber
4. Balanced and varied

Now who is going to argue with that??

Put the Target on your refrigerator. Practice eating from all four groups shooting for the bull's-eye as much as possible. When an occasional arrow hits the outer circle, let it fall without guilt or remorse. Of course, if you stray off center too often, return to the basic guidelines.

Ben Franklin once said that his best inventions were often the simplest; that is, the result of years of work can be a surprisingly simple product. The Target idea appears simple, but it has a lot of power. Putting four simple rules into a target diagram solves many other nutrition concerns. The Target helps you memorize and picture the four fundamental principles of eating. Once you learn these, you will be amazed how readily they provide answers to most of the other nutrition questions that come up. It's like elementary math versus calculus. No matter how sophisticated the calculus problem, it won't get solved if the mathematician forgets that two plus two equals four.

Let me add some fine points to the Smart Eating Food Target so you can put its power to work for you.

Eat, drink, but be wary — for tomorrow you may live!

3

Expanding the Target

ONCE YOU GRASP the principle of the Smart Eating Food Target, you can easily expand it to include every food.

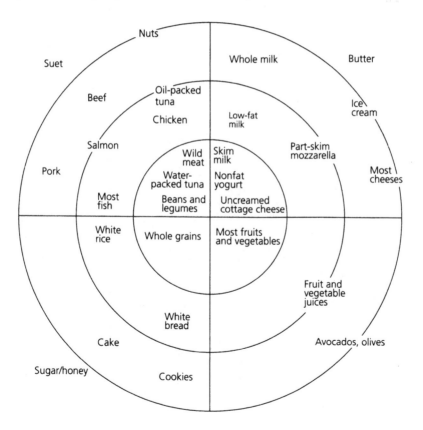

I rank foods in the milk group by their fat content. Skim (or nonfat) milk goes in the center ring, since it has no fat at all. Milk with 1 percent fat is next to the skim, 2 percent low-fat milk is in the next ring, and "regular" (whole) milk, which is 3.5 percent, is in the outer ring. That's confusing, isn't it? How can something that has only 3.5 percent fat be in the outer ring? Here's the reason. Whole milk is about 87 percent calorie-free water, 3.5 percent fat, and about 9.5 percent protein and carbohydrate. All the calories are in the fat, protein, and carbohydrates, so even though the fat is 3.5 percent *by volume,* it provides 72 of the 160 calories in the glass. That means 45 percent of the calories are fat calories. Bottom line — 3.5 percent milk by volume is 45 percent fat calories!

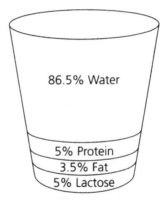

As we continue adding milk-group foods to the Target, the amounts of fat are less obvious. Cheese, in particular, fools a lot of people. Some cheeses are fairly low in fat, such as low-fat and non-fat cottage cheese and part-skim mozzarella, but most cheeses (all the ones I like!) are way out on the outer circles of the Target. Luckily the food manufacturers must be listening to our needs, because new low-fat cheeses are showing up in the markets every day.

And then there's ice cream. The really good ice creams are about 60 percent fat calories. But — it's okay to eat them because they have medicinal value. Everyone knows that ice cream cures depression. For children it's an analgesic — it takes away pain instantly. I'm joking, of course — be careful not to let too many stray arrows hit the ice cream ring.

What about butter? Butter is so far removed from milk that I've put it outside the Target. Like lard, margarine, vegetable oils, and mayonnaise, butter is pure fat and contains virtually no vitamins, minerals, or protein. It isn't a food at all — it's grease extracted from a food.

Let's move on to the meat group, which is also arranged according to fat content, with beans and other legumes located near the bull's-eye, beef in the middle ring, and bacon at the outer edge. In some ways vegetarians are smarter than meat eaters because they eat lots of low-fat, high-fiber beans, thereby getting meat-group nutrition but avoiding the fat inherent in most meats. Unfortunately, some vegetarians are not so smart. They get their meat nutrients from tofu or eggs, both of which are 60 percent fat calories. Even worse are the vegetarians who eat nuts or seeds for their meat nutrients, for nuts and seeds are not much more than fat encased in a shell. You won't find a nut with less than 78 percent fat calories! If you're a vegetarian, watch where you aim your arrows when you make selections from the meat group.

Where does fish go on the Target? If it isn't doctored up with butter or creamy sauces, most fish is close to the bull's-eye. Water-packed tuna, for instance, is less than 10 percent fat calories; pack it in oil and you have 37 percent fat calories. Notice that salmon is in the same ring with oil-drenched tuna. Yes, all by itself, with no sauces added, salmon is 35–40 percent fat.

Game meat gets a thumbs-up on the Target. Deer, rabbit, and quail are all low in fat. My rule is: if it runs, it's lean, so eat it!

I used to put all pork outside of the Target, but pig farmers, listening to society's demands, are now producing a leaner product. Bacon and sausage are still on the outer edge of the Target, but the other cuts are usually comparable to beef in fat content. I put suet on the diagram mostly for fun, but keep in mind that suet is pure grease separated from meat, just as butter is pure grease extracted from milk.

Everything below the center line is graded by its fiber content, which you can think of as its "wholeness" or "whole-grainness," that is, how close it is to its natural state when eaten. Cake is made of wheat flour, just as whole-wheat bread is, but whole-wheat flour is much closer to the natural wheat than highly refined white cake flour.

In the bread and cereal group, whole grains go in the bull's-eye. Whole grain means unrefined, unbleached — in short, untouched. Some health-food nuts pull whole wheat apart and sprinkle bran on their cereal or mix wheat germ into their milkshakes. That's okay, but I urge people to eat whole wheat because it has more trace minerals than refined bran, wheat, and wheat germ eaten separately. In this case, the whole is greater than the sum of its parts.

In contrast, the *caloric* value of wheat is lower than that of the sum of its parts. As part of whole wheat, bran makes the starch less digestible, so the caloric value of whole-wheat bread is lower than the charts usually show. A pound of white bread has more calories and less nutrition than a pound of whole-wheat bread because the carbohydrate becomes more digestible when the bran is removed. The same is true for rice, corn, rye, millet, oats, and any other grain you can think of. A cup of cornstarch will make you a lot fatter than a cup of corn kernels. What a shame it is that we deliberately alter cereal grains so that the vitamin/mineral content goes down, the fiber content goes down, and the caloric content goes up. We seem determined to make our foods less nutritious.

Sugar and honey, like butter and suet, do not belong inside the Target — they are completely devoid of vitamins and minerals. This statement rankles some "health conscious" people who claim that honey has a few trace minerals and therefore is more nutritious than sugar. They're right, of course. Honey has a tiny, tiny amount of minerals — you only need a cup of honey to equal the minerals in a forkful of cake! Get my point? Don't kid yourself that either sugar or honey is better than the other.

The last food group — fruits and vegetables — is the easiest to discuss because almost all fruits and vegetables are low in fat, low in calories, and high in fiber. Except for avocados and olives, which have a lot of fat, all of them go in the bull's-eye, unless you juice them (see p. 10).

It should be obvious that very fat people should eat from the bull's-eye only. Someone who is less fat can add foods from the next ring, and the very fit can get away with some selections from the outer ring.

If you select most of your food from the center rings of the Target you can bring about many of the dietary changes that experts recommend. Using Target principles to make food choices eliminates the need for trendy diet books, protein drinks, and vitamin supplements. More important, choosing foods wisely can significantly improve the health of those suffering from diabetes, recovering from heart attacks, or just plain fighting obesity. If you eat smart, most of your dietary worries will be over.

4

And There Are Fringe Benefits!

WHEN YOU EAT using Target principles, most of your other nutrition concerns will be satisfied without extra effort. Cholesterol, for example, is usually associated with animal fats and is therefore found only in the outer circles of the meat and milk groups. As you move toward the center of the Target, cholesterol decreases automatically. Bull's-eye foods, having no cholesterol at all, are the foods that heart patients are urged to eat. Shellfish are an exception; they are located near the center of the Target because they are low in fat, but they are slightly higher in cholesterol. The Target doesn't require the eater to think about cholesterol, because a diet that is low in fat is automatically low in cholesterol.

What about saturated (animal) versus polyunsaturated (vegetable) fats? In the past we were told that unsaturated fats are better, but recent studies linking certain kinds of cancer to unsaturated fats suggest that this may not be true. A simple solution is to take the Target approach, which automatically decreases the total fat in your diet. When total dietary fat is low enough, the type of fat becomes relatively insignificant.

Another advantage of the Target approach is that your intake of food additives is automatically reduced. This is particularly obvious in the breads and cereals category. Packaged cakes, cookies, and pastries contain staggering amounts of preservatives. Food dyes, stabilizers, texturizers, flavor enhancers all show up in sugar-rich, fiber-poor packaged breads and cereals. The more natural and fiber-rich the grain product, the fewer the additives. In the meat and milk groups, the levels of food additives rise as the fat level goes up. As you move toward the center of the Target the purity of the foods increases, another healthy spinoff of low-fat, low-sugar, high-fiber eating.

Perhaps the greatest advantage of eating from the center of the Target is the sharp increase in your diet's nutrient content, or nutrient density. On the Target the nutrients *per calorie* rise as you approach the bull's-eye. It's true that a glass of whole milk contains the same amount of vitamins, minerals, and protein as a glass of skim milk, but the whole milk contains twice as many calories because of its fat content. In the old days whole milk was considered nutritious because of its many nutrients. Now we understand that whole milk isn't nutritious because its nutrition *per calorie* is too low. If you drink two glasses of skim milk, you get the same number of calories as you do from one glass of whole milk, but you get twice the vitamins, minerals, and protein.

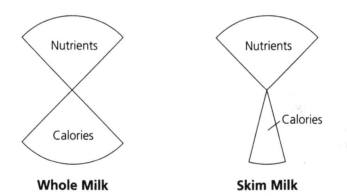

Whole Milk   **Skim Milk**

Eating from the center of the Target ensures that your diet will be high in nutrient density and you won't consume too many calories. If — and this is a big if — you eat predominantly bull's-eye foods, it is a waste of money to take vitamin/mineral supplements. If, on the other hand, you eat from the four food groups, but your selections are white bread, French-fried zucchini, whole milk, and bacon, you will not only be vitamin/mineral deficient but you will also get fat! As you get fatter, you may eat less, but if you continue to make the same poor selections, you'll get fewer vitamins and minerals.

The people in the United States who have marginal vitamin deficiencies shouldn't blame the problem on foods grown in poor soil or on slow shipping and handling. These deficiencies are caused by the low-nutrient, high-fat, high-sugar foods that they eat. Put the blame where it belongs — not on the farmer, the food handlers, or the markets but squarely on the eater! Don't claim our supermarket foods have no nutrients if you eat hot dogs and potato chips and put vitamin-free margarine on your bread.

The Target has several other spinoff advantages. Foods at the center tend to be low in salt (although this advantage can be negated at the dinner table). Bull's-eye foods usually cost less, and supermarket prices are high enough to make economy important to all of us. Also, many foods from the center of the Target last well in storage. Grains of edible wheat were discovered when King Tut's tomb was opened, and potatoes buried with the Inca Indians have been found to be edible. Beans stored simply in bags can last for years. People in poorer countries without modern refrigeration and storage facilities owe their existence to grains and legumes.

I started this discussion of the Target by claiming that you need to obey only four dietary rules. You can now see that the Target principles, based on these four rules, actually provide for most of today's other dietary requisites as well. Foods from the center of the target are:

• low in fat	• low in saturated fats
• low in sugar	• low in cost
• low in calories	• highly storable
• low in salt	• high in fiber
• low in additives	• high in vitamins
• low in cholesterol	• high in minerals
• high in protein	• a balanced diet

5

Going for Quantity

THE CALORIES in a half cup of peanuts equal the calories in six baked potatoes. Stop a moment, close your eyes, and think about what you just read. Picture a man holding a half cup of peanuts in one hand — and a can of beer in the other to wash them down. Now picture the same man trying to hold six potatoes in one hand! Most men can wolf down a handful of peanuts and not think twice about it. But who's going to wolf down six potatoes?

"But," you say, "when I want a snack, I'm not thinking potatoes." Okay, instead of grabbing a handful of peanuts (and wishing for more) eat a big bag of popcorn (hold the butter, please). It takes *sixteen cups* of popcorn to equal the calories in that measly handful of peanuts.

I like the Target principles because they allow me to eat a lot of food. For the same number of calories I can have two cups of skim milk instead of one cup of whole milk. A big bowl of split-pea soup with a thick slice of whole-wheat bread is equivalent in calories to a fast-food hamburger but far more filling. I can have two or three oranges instead of one glass of orange juice.

People who have previously tried dieting are amazed at how much food the Target approach allows. In fact, they often complain that we expect them to eat too much food. You like chicken? Eat a chicken breast with the skin on it and you get 15 grams of fat. Remove the skin and you cut it to 8 grams of fat. My greedy mind says that means I can have another piece of chicken!

Doughnuts are deep-fried disasters. In just a few bites you consume 360 calories, including 11 grams (that's more than two teaspoons) of fat. For the same calorie count, but only 3 grams of fat, you could have *six* slices of whole-wheat toast with fruit spread and nonfat cream cheese. I can gobble a doughnut in seconds, but *six* slices of toast would slow even me down.

I like to eat! I like to eat often and I like to eat a lot of food. Sometimes I stray to the perimeter of the Target, but most of the time I aim for the center because I can go for quantity. People desperate to lose weight yearn for a secret new combination of foods, but they're overlooking the rules that have been here forever. They wouldn't have gained weight in the first place if they had eaten according to the Target, and they can lose weight if they start now to follow the Target. If you use the Target principles, YOU WILL HAVE NO FEELING OF DENIAL AT ALL.

6

A Picture in My Mind

MY TARGET APPROACH is powerful because it allows you to be who you are. It allows *you* to design *your own* diet. It gives you tools to plan and coordinate meals as much — or as little — as your temperament demands.

If you're the plan-ahead type, you can plan every food and meal to the last tiny detail using the Target rules. You can even cook a week's menus in advance, freeze them, and enjoy ready-made home-cooked meals every night.

Or you might be more like me. I never plan anything. I'm one of those people who can't remember what I ate at my last meal no matter how good it was. I have absolutely no idea what I'm going to eat at my next meal. But in spite of my apparent lack of interest in food planning, I'm always conscious of the four basic Target rules when I eat.

When I'm out to dinner at a friend's home or a restaurant, I mentally superimpose a target over my plate, sliding food around to see if I can account for all the food groups. I even draw those concentric rings in my mind, mentally shifting foods by their fat, fiber, and sugar content.

The Target principles help me to eat smart, getting all my vitamins from low-fat, low-sugar foods. I don't need to carry thick books on nutrition or pocket food guides. I don't have to carry anything with me EXCEPT — a picture in my mind.

7

Rapid Weight Loss

THE TARGET PRINCIPLES don't rely on counting calories or reading lists of forbidden foods. They simply rely on your mental picture of food values. If you mentally "target" your meals, you will achieve and maintain your ideal weight. But what if you have gained a lot of weight? You want to do more than eat smart. You want to drop some fat NOW.

Add fat-gram counting to your regimen. It really helps!

Notice that the chart on page 25 gives three possible selections for each goal weight. The choice depends on how quickly you want to lose fat. If you are super-eager, choose the 10 percent column, but I must warn you — a 10-percent-fat diet is stringent and difficult to follow. If you're willing to accept a longer-term weight-loss goal, choose the 20 percent column. And if you're close to or already at your ideal weight, use the 25 percent column.

Suppose a 300-pound person desperately wants to weigh 150 pounds. By using my method, he cuts fat intake drastically but continues to get the nutrients he needs by eating heartily from the inner rings of the Target. He should begin by dropping back two levels on the chart, consuming no more than 40 grams of fat a day (which is the amount in the 10 percent column for a 280-pound person). When his weight gets to 280 pounds he should then reduce his fat intake to 38 grams (the 10-percent column for 260 pounds) and so on until he reaches his desired weight.

Notice that I don't mention how many calories to eat. When you cut way back on fat, you have to eat A LOT of food for the calories to add up. True, some people can get too many calories on a 10-percent-fat diet, but that requires a lot of eating. On a 10-percent-fat

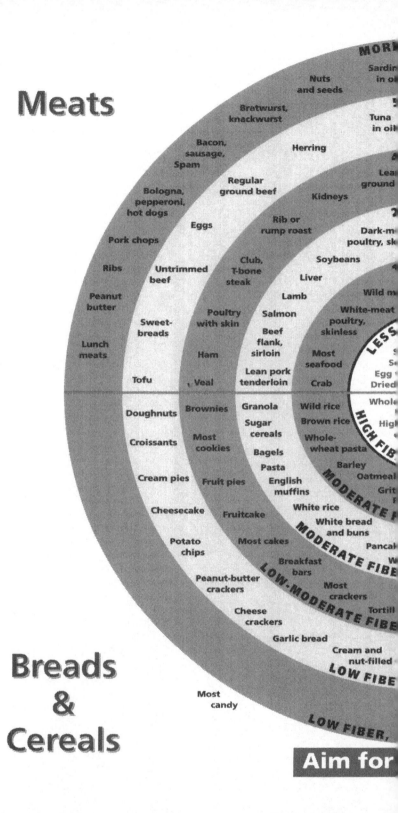

Meats

Breads & Cereals

MOR[...]

Sardin[es]
in oi[l]

Nuts
and seeds

Bratwurst,
knackwurst

Tuna
in oil

Bacon,
sausage,
Spam

Herring

Lea[n]
ground

Bologna,
pepperoni,
hot dogs

Regular
ground beef

Kidneys

Eggs

Rib or
rump roast

Dark-m[eat]
poultry, sk[in]

Pork chops

Soybeans

Ribs

Untrimmed
beef

Club,
T-bone
steak

Liver

Wild m[eat]

Peanut
butter

Lamb

White-meat
poultry,
skinless

Sweet-
breads

Poultry
with skin

Salmon

Beef
flank,
sirloin

Most
seafood

LES[S]

Lunch
meats

Ham

S[...]
S[...]

Tofu

Veal

Lean pork
tenderloin

Crab

Egg [...]
Dried

Whol[e]

Doughnuts

Brownies

Granola

Wild rice

Hig[h]

Sugar
cereals

Brown rice

Croissants

Most
cookies

Whole-
wheat pasta

HIGH FIB[ER]

Bagels

Barley

Cream pies

Fruit pies

Pasta

English
muffins

Oatmeal

Grit[s]

Cheesecake

Fruitcake

White rice

MODERATE [...]

Potato
chips

Most cakes

White bread
and buns

Pancak[es]

MODERATE FIBE[R]

Breakfast
bars

W[...]

Peanut-butter
crackers

Most
crackers

LOW-MODERATE FIBE[R]

Cheese
crackers

Tortill[a]

LOW-MODERATE FIBE[R]

Garlic bread

Cream and
nut-filled

LOW FIBE[R]

Most
candy

LOW FIBER,

Aim for

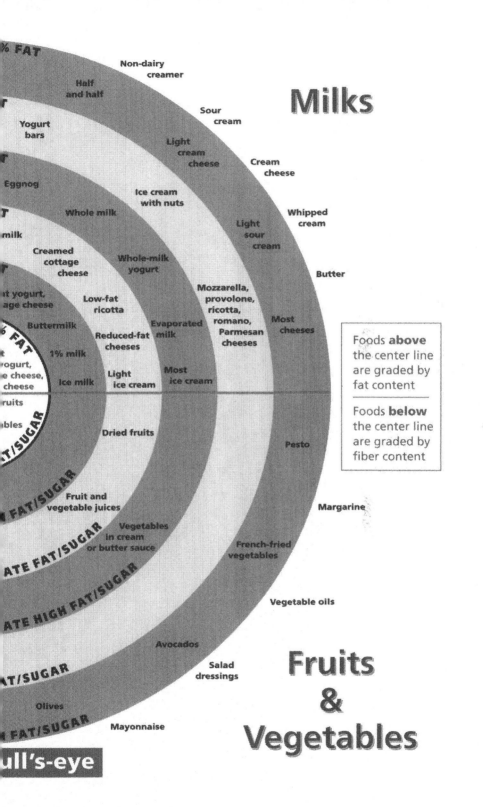

Milks

Non-dairy creamer

Half and half

Yogurt bars

Sour cream

Eggnog

Light cream cheese

Cream cheese

Whole milk

Ice cream with nuts

Whipped cream

milk

Light sour cream

Creamed cottage cheese

Whole-milk yogurt

Butter

t yogurt, age cheese

Low-fat ricotta

Mozzarella, provolone, ricotta, romano, Parmesan cheeses

Buttermilk

Evaporated milk

Most cheeses

yogurt, e cheese, cheese

Reduced-fat cheeses

1% milk

Ice milk

Light ice cream

Most ice cream

ruits

ables

Foods **above** the center line are graded by fat content

Foods **below** the center line are graded by fiber content

Dried fruits

Pesto

Fruit and vegetable juices

Vegetables in cream or butter sauce

Margarine

French-fried vegetables

Vegetable oils

Avocados

Salad dressings

Fruits & Vegetables

Olives

Mayonnaise

ull's-eye

Recommended Daily Grams of Fat

	Percentage of Fat in Diet				Percentage of Fat in Diet		
	25%	**20%**	**10%**		**25%**	**20%**	**10%**
Goal Weight	*do not need to lose weight*	*need to lose less than 25 pounds*	*need to lose more than 25 pounds*	**Goal Weight**	*do not need to lose weight*	*need to lose less than 25 pounds*	*need to lose more than 25 pounds*
100 lbs.	36 g	29 g	14 g	210 lbs.	76 g	61 g	30 g
110	40	32	16	220	79	64 g	32
120	43	35	17	230	83	66 g	33
130	47	38	19	240	87	69 g	35
140	50	40	20	250	90	72 g	36
150	54	43	22	260	94	75 g	38
160	58	46	23	270	98	78 g	39
170	61	49	25	280	101	81	40
180	65	52	26	290	105	84	42
190	69	55	27	300	108	87	43
200	72	58	29	310	112	90	45

HOW TO USE THIS CHART

If you do not need to lose weight:
Find your actual weight in the Goal Weight column and follow the recommendation for the 25% fat diet. The grams listed are based on a somewhat sedentary lifestyle. If you are exercising moderately, you can eat 5–10 grams of fat above the recommended number.

If you want to lose less than 25 pounds:
Find the "goal weight" you want to achieve and follow the recommendation for the 20% fat diet. When you have reached your desired weight, switch to the 25% fat diet.

If you want to lose more than 25 pounds:
IMPORTANT! Do not use the recommendation for your goal weight, because the difference between that and your current weight may be too drastic. Instead, find a goal weight 20 pounds below your current weight and follow the recommendation for the 10% fat diet. When you have achieved that goal weight, drop 20 more pounds and again follow the recommendation for the 10% fat diet. When you are within 25 pounds of your desired weight, switch to the recommendation for the 20% fat diet. When you have reached your desired weight, switch to the 25% fat diet.

diet most rational people get full long before they consume too many calories.

Some of my readers don't need to lose weight — but they need to watch their fat intake for medical reasons. If you are at high risk for a heart attack or have high blood cholesterol or dangerous blood-triglyceride levels, counting grams of fat is a must for you. In most cases your physician or dietitian would recommend the 10 percent level called for in the famous Pritikin Diet. I urge you to follow my chart, using the 10 percent column. You can tell your friends you are on the Pritikin Diet or — you can tell them you are "on Target."

Whether you use the chart as a guideline for weight loss, for health reasons, or simply for fat intake, I must caution you about one thing. Charts like mine that recommend grams of fat can be misused if you focus so much on fat that you forget the common-sense rules of smart eating. For example, if you ate only jelly beans, you would be on a zero-percent-fat diet — and you would die of malnutrition. If you avoided *all* meats instead of avoiding only the high-fat meats on the Target's periphery, you would indeed lower your fat intake — but you might also become deficient in iron.

In other words, counting grams of fat should not be a goal in itself, it should be done in addition to following the Target principles. DO NOT do one without the other.

EACH DAY YOU SHOULD NOT, UNDER ANY CIRCUMSTANCES EAT LESS THAN:

> Two foods from the meat group
> Two foods from the milk group
> Four foods from breads and cereals
> Four foods from fruits and vegetables

These are minimums! Obviously, a large person with a higher goal weight will eat more food, quickly exceeding those minimums. The ratio, however, should stay about the same; that is, you should try to eat twice as many nonanimal foods (the lower half of the Target) as meat- and milk-group foods (upper half of the Target). As your consumption of food and calories rises, it is wise to increase the servings of whole-wheat breads and cereals and high-fiber fruits and vegetables rather than the meats and milks.

Notice that this approach keeps a check on your consumption of animal foods, but in a balanced and positive way. Instead of omitting these foods altogether, as some radical diets recommend, my method recognizes the high vitamin, mineral, and protein content of meats and milks, then urges you to make low-fat selections. Now isn't that calm and rational?

Counting fat grams is very popular now, and tables similar to mine can be found in many books. My method, however, is unique because:

1. You start with Target principles. You don't focus on counting fat until you understand and know how to use the Target rules.
2. You can increase the fat in your diet as you approach your goal weight.
3. You select your correct daily fat intake based on your desired weight. Other programs often recommend:
   a. an average amount, such as 50 grams a day, for everyone, as if we all had the same needs. Or
   b. fat grams based on your current weight instead of your *goal* weight. Or
   c. fat intake based on the number of pounds you need to lose.

Naturally I think my method is the best, but let's face it. What's the *real* value of counting grams of fat? It isn't in meeting a precise number each day. It's that the process of counting and looking up fat grams on labels and in books makes people *aware* of what they are eating. Even people who think they are nutrition-conscious are surprised when they learn just how much fat their favorite foods contain.

Daily Caloric Requirements*

The recommendations for daily grams of fat (page 25) are based on these caloric requirements for a "sedentary" person. Naturally, if you exercise moderately, these numbers should be higher. Suppose, for example, my recommendation for you is 50 grams of fat. If you exercise every day, you can increase that number by 5–10 grams. Even people who need to make a drastic reduction in fat intake can occasionally get away with eating 3–5 extra grams if they exercise regularly.

Goal Weight	Caloric Requirements	Goal Weight	Caloric Requirements
100 lbs.	1300 cal./day	210 lbs.	2730 cal./day
110	1430	220	2860
120	1560	230	2990
130	1690	240	3120
140	1820	250	3250
150	1950	260	3380
160	2080	270	3510
170	2210	280	3640
180	2340	290	3770
190	2470	300	3900
200	2600	310	4030

*Based on the formula: weight × 13 = recommended daily calories. Please don't focus on calorie intake. This chart is mainly intended for those scientific types who want to know how I calculated the recommended grams of fat in Table 1.

8

Making Foods Wet

LOW-FAT EATING generates one legitimate complaint: the foods seem dry! It's a funny expression really, because fats and oils aren't wet at all. If you put Vaseline on your hands, would you say your hands feel wet? We put butter on toast so it won't be so dry, even though butter is a grease, which doesn't make the toast wet. It makes the toast greasy.

Semantics aside, taking fat and oil out of our diet makes foods seem dry. Potatoes, formerly lavished with butter and sour cream, are awfully hard to swallow when dry. I, for one, have not mastered the art of eating a baked potato with nothing on it. Dry toast with no butter or jelly also seems hard to choke down. It's too dry. As we take the fat out of our diet, more and more foods become dry and somehow less satisfying.

My solution is to make foods wet. As you reduce the fat replace it with water. I'm not suggesting you pour a cup of water over your toast or your baked potato, but dunking toast in your coffee or tea isn't that different, is it?

A good way to make foods wet is to use lots of tomatoes (canned ones in winter). After all, a tomato is nothing more than a bag of red water that doesn't spill when you slice it! We put chopped tomatoes on baked potatoes just before serving. We put sliced tomatoes in sandwiches in place of mayonnaise and butter. We put tomatoes on pasta and eat cherry tomatoes as snacks. Tomatoes are a miracle food!

Here's a trick. The next time you eat out, order a baked potato (be sure the chef doesn't put anything on it) and a salad without dressing. Open the potato and dump the salad all over it. The water in the lettuce, tomatoes, and other vegetables makes the potato wet, so you don't need any butter and sour cream. If that's not wet enough for you, add a nonfat salad dressing. I especially like a nonfat ranch or blue-cheese dressing on potatoes.

Cottage cheese is wet! We put the low-fat variety on practically everything, even a dollop in the middle of a spicy-hot chili.

Traditional gravies are so filled with fat that conscientious low-fat eaters won't touch them. But heat up chicken or beef broth with some low-fat evaporated milk, a teaspoon of Butter Buds, mixed with a little cornstarch, herbs, and some garlic or onion powder, and you've got a tasty low-fat gravy. And gravies are terrific for making foods wet. By doing it right, you can have mashed potatoes and gravy again. You see, it IS possible to feast without guilt!

When I was a boy, my mom occasionally heated a can of lima beans for lunch, poured out the water, and served them dry on a plate with other foods. I could not swallow those lima beans. I hated them. Then one day she didn't pour out the water. She served the limas with their watery juices in a bowl, to be eaten with a spoon. I loved them! Adding water prompted the total turnaround of a stubborn kid in ten minutes.

Soup, perhaps, is our ultimate wet-food achievement. I could live on soup! It fills you up without filling you out. By dipping into the pot deep or shallow you can have your soup thick or thin. If you can't think what to do with some tired vegetables, make minestrone. If kidney beans or red beans seem too dry, make them into bean soup. Soups not only make food wet that would otherwise be dry, they also usually contain foods from three or four of the groups, yielding a balanced meal in a bowl. If your soup has foods from three groups but no milk-group food, add cottage cheese. Be sure the soup is hot and put the cottage cheese on the table so that people can help themselves. Cold cottage cheese in hot soup. Perfect!

I used to guide weeklong canoe trips in Canada. I had to plan the menus very carefully ahead of time because people eat a lot of food outdoors and we couldn't afford the weight of extra supplies. To make sure we didn't run out of food in the middle of the trip, I served soup before every lunch and every dinner. The dry soup mixes weighed next to nothing in our packs, but cooked with lots of lake water, they allowed people to fill up before eating our precious solid foods.

Getting people to eat less by filling them up with soup is a sensible restaurateur's trick. Restaurant chefs don't have to worry about weight the way I did, but they know how to slow our hunger with inexpensive soups so that we are satisfied with smaller portions of their expensive main courses.

Wow! Adding liquid to foods should be a fifth Target rule! It not only makes dry foods more palatable, it helps to fill you up so you won't be tempted to turn to high-fat, high-sugar foods.

9

Athletes — Breaking the Target Rules

ATHLETES! LISTEN UP! Don't take antisugar or anticarbohydrate advice from fat friends or fat researchers. You may have seen recent newspaper articles reporting that carbohydrates are more fattening than we originally thought — that fat people quickly gain weight on carbohydrates. Well, of course they do. If you're overweight and out of shape, your muscles require more insulin to get glucose into the muscle. Carbohydrate that doesn't get into the muscle is converted to fat. I described the physiology of the insulin response to dietary carbohydrate in *Fit or Fat?* in 1975. In other words, more than twenty years ago I was telling fat people not to eat sugar because their high insulin response would drive sugar into their fat cells.

As usual, the news people aren't printing news. Carbohydrates ARE fattening — for fat people. Athletes, on the other hand, produce very little insulin when they eat pasta, bread, potatoes, or simple sugars. Their muscles absorb the sugar from these foods readily, and later those same muscles burn up the stored sugars. In fact, the athlete's need to store and use sugar in muscle is so great that for one hour after long, intense exercise, pure simple sugar is their food of choice.

CARBOHYDRATES
ARE
FATTENING
for FAT people.

CARBOHYDRATES
ARE NOT
FATTENING
for FIT people.

During that hour after exercise (sometimes called the glycogen window), an athlete's muscles desperately suck up all available sugar to replace their depleted glycogen. Sports drinks are usually the quickest way to accomplish this, but *any* sugar will work, even a bowl of Jell-O. Candy bars would also do the trick, but they're full of fat. Don't think for a minute that a Power Bar after exercise is magical. Its only magic is that its number-one ingredient is sugar. Right after exercise you don't need all those "magical" vitamins and minerals — you need sugar!

Being an athlete gives you an advantage, doesn't it? You get to fudge (pun intended) one of the four Target rules — you can have sugar now and then.

Pay attention, however, to my rule *Eat Less Fat*. Long-distance athletes really prosper on a lower in fat diet. After digestion and absorption, fat from food appears in the blood as a milky white substance. It causes red blood cells to clump together, slowing their passage through the capillaries and delaying the delivery of oxygen. For six to eight hours after a fatty meal, a well-trained runner experiences a significant drop in performance. Fatty, clumped blood moves slowly, so the heart has to pump harder. An athlete may not notice that the heart is working harder, but imagine the effect on the weak heart of a nonathlete.

I bet you thought I wouldn't admit to a shortcoming of the Target principles. Well, there is one. Long-distance runners not only use protein to build tissues (like the rest of us), they also burn up a lot of protein as fuel (most of us do not do this). Additionally, long-distance running breaks down red blood cells, and the runners lose iron, which often makes them anemic.

The need for protein is easily handled by the Target because it allows these athletes to eat lots of food. Trust me, if they eat a lot they WILL get more than enough protein. It's possible, however, that their need for iron may not be met by basic Target eating. This is especially true if they eat a lot of carbohydrates, which are low in iron. If athletes eat a bit more meat than I normally recommend, they can still prosper on the Target plan. But if they follow the popular antimeat sentiment, avoiding even low-fat meats, they must take iron supplements.

Now, after all that, let's rewrite the four rules for athletes because obviously they have special needs. An athlete should have a diet that is:

1. Low in fat
2. Low in sugar — except after strenuous exercise
3. High in fiber
4. Balanced and varied — with plenty of food.

Not so different from the basics, huh? Whether you're fit or fat, the rules are pretty much the same. Athletes just get to bend the rules more. They're allowed to have sugar now and then (rule no. 2), and they get to eat LOTS more food (rule no. 4).

10

Natural Vitamins

PEOPLE OFTEN ASK ME, "Do you believe in natural vitamins?" What a silly question. That's like asking if I believe in clean air or pure water. Of course I believe in natural vitamins.

What I DON'T believe is that we need to have those vitamins manufactured for us in pill form. Taking little pills every day is the most unnatural way I can think of to get your vitamins. Even the expression "natural vitamin pill" is absurd. It's like military intelligence and jumbo shrimp. Calling pills in little bottles "natural vitamins" is the ultimate oxymoron. Good nutrition doesn't come from pills. The vitamin salesmen who tell you the key to good health comes from a bottle are selling you a hoax. Don't buy into the scam!

No one would argue that sitting around, NOT EXERCISING, is an insult to our muscles. They are designed to be worked, and we've all seen the results if muscles are not used — flabby, unattractive bodies, obesity, frailty in old age.

Nor would anyone disagree with the notion that our brains are meant to be used. There is intriguing research showing that the more we challenge ourselves with problem-solving, the more we develop intricate and varied nerve connections in the brain. Apparently, actively using your brain when you're young allows it to stay active when you're old.

Even bones thrive on being used. Studies have shown that people who are active have denser bones than those who are sedentary. The osteoporosis of old age can be largely prevented or delayed if you exercise a lot.

The heart, lungs, kidneys, liver — *every* organ and tissue in your body prospers from being worked and does poorly when not used. Why, then, do you insult your digestive system by not using it? The intestines were meant to work! They're *supposed* to break down food and extract vitamins! They like it when you eat high-fiber food — it challenges them. When you dump a bunch of manufactured pills in your body, the intestines say, "Humph! I guess she doesn't want me to work anymore." Challenge them! Eat lots of high-fiber foods and say to your intestines, "You'll really have to work to get the vitamins out of this!"

People who feel they need vitamin pills often also have a very strong natural-foods bent. They grind fresh peanuts for additive-free peanut butter. They go for goat's milk and cheeses to avoid the extensive pasteurization and other processing of cow's milk. They were among the first to advocate the return to whole grains. Their avoidance of food preservatives, chemicals, and stabilizers parallels their abhorrence of alcohol and drugs. In other words, these people are at the forefront of the health movement. And yet they take vitamin pills, factory-made and totally unnatural. What a paradox.

The word "vitamin" means a nutrient, essential for life, found in microscopic amounts in food.

Learn to get your vitamins the SMART WAY — from food!

11

What about the Kids?

I'M ONE OF THE LUCKIEST MEN on earth. My two children are now healthy adults. They're physically active, have low body fat, live life to its fullest, and have meaningful relationships. They don't smoke, drink, or use drugs. What did their mother and I do that contributed to those results? If I knew the answer, I would be advising parents how to raise children instead of how to exercise and eat sensibly.

So when well-meaning parents ask, "What about my kids? How can I get them to exercise and eat well?" I tell them the only thing I know — to practice what they preach.

My children grew up in an environment in which activity and adventures were natural parts of life. We climbed mountains, skied, biked, and went swimming every chance we got. We didn't park the kids in front of the television to keep them busy, and we didn't serve them high-fat frozen dinners to save us time. Food was not the focus of our existence but a way to get fuel for the next soccer game or square dance outing. When we snacked we didn't worry that the foods were filled with saturated fats because we ate a low-fat diet. Fitness and good health were no big deal — just a way of life.

Make sure your kids know the four basic rules and how to apply them with the Target. When our children were very young, we cut pictures of food from magazines and glued them on a big target on the wall. The kids were soon teaching the Target principles to our neighbors. As they got older we graduated to placemats with the Target on them. I had visions of Target placemats and Target wall posters becoming as popular as Hula Hoops and pet rocks.

Worried about your children's health? Don't sit on the sidelines. Get up and set an example by exercising. Just do it — and your kids will do it too!

12

The Power of the Four Rules

THE MOST POWERFUL THING you can learn from this book is that the Target principles will last forever. Believe them and apply them every day of your life and you will never again be confused by nutrition advice. When newspaper articles or well-intentioned friends assault you with the latest nutrition "miracle," evaluate that new concept to see if it violates any of the four unbendable Target rules.

When, for example, I first heard of the supposed wonders of fish oils, with their miraculous omega-3 fatty acids, I was able to put the information in context immediately. Fish oils are oils; that is, they are liquid fat. While omega-3 fatty acids have interesting pharmacological properties, they are nonetheless fat. It's not smart eating to purchase quantities of them to pour over a well-balanced low-fat diet.

Some years ago a campaign was launched to convince Americans to avoid saturated fats and substitute polyunsaturated fats in their place. The purveyors of the idea meant well, for excellent studies had been done proving that saturated fats were likely to end up in artery walls and precipitate heart attacks. But people got the impression that polyunsaturated fats were actually *good* for them rather than simply *less bad*. As a result, fat consumption in America actually increased! What's the Target rule? *Eat Less Fat*, be it oil, margarine, or bacon grease. If it feels greasy on your fingers, avoid it, even if it's polyunsaturated. If your mechanic can grease your car with it, don't eat it.

There used to be a popular diet — guaranteed to burn fat — in which you ate nothing but fruit day in and day out. That's low fat, isn't it? It's also high fiber and fairly low sugar. It sounded good to lots of people, but it violated the "balanced diet" rule. So it was not a good diet.

What about the people who say that humans are the only animals that drink milk after they are weaned and you should never, ever drink milk? Are they breaking a Target rule? In a similar vein, some people extol the virtues of eating just one food to the exclusion of others, like the once popular macrobiotic rice diet. They're both breaking grandma's rule, aren't they? Eat a balanced diet!

Here's a fun one for you. Which rule is broken by those fast-weight-loss liquid diets that claim to have all the vitamins you need? No fiber, right? Not to mention all those "fake" vitamins that are added. You think your intestines are going to enjoy that?

Nutrition isn't confusing when you follow the Target principles. In fact it gets to be fun. I get weirdo questions all the time about one diet or another, and I answer by applying the four rules. If any rule is violated, I throw out the diet!

If you want to sort out the truth about conflicting nutrition advice, use the four rules. They work every time.

13

The Miracle of Food

WHO WOULD HAVE KNOWN seventy-five years ago that cutting down trees in our forests would affect the fish in the streams and the ozone layer surrounding our planet? Trees provide so many useful products, harvesting them seemed a natural and wonderful way to have a better life. Inevitably many things were harmed by a seemingly innocent pursuit.

We have such a hunger for secret cures — for something new and "magical" that will change us and improve our health that we've done the same thing with food. In trying to improve our lifestyle we've often destroyed the natural way in which food is meant to be eaten.

Rice, once eaten by millions in its crude form, was refined into white rice. At first a rich man's food, white rice eventually became the *only* food for vast millions of people in the Orient, precipitating a host of medical problems, including protein deficiencies and beriberi.

The story is repeated with the refinement of flour. For centuries everyone ate whole-wheat bread. Then the technology for milling and refining flour produced white bread. Because it was expensive it was called the "king's bread." Peasants clamored for it, not realizing that white flour lacks a host of vitamins and minerals, especially B vitamins. They eventually got the riches formerly reserved for the king — including his vitamin-B deficiency.

At the turn of the century nutritionists observed widespread malnutrition among poorer Americans. They attributed it to a lack of protein and B vitamins, the nutrients found mainly in meats and other animal products. A great campaign began for people to eat more meat, which they did. Malnutrition rates subsided, but more and more people got heart attacks. It took nutritionists far too long to comprehend that the diet they had pushed was too high in fat and cholesterol.

Now the pendulum has swung away from animal products. People eat fruits and vegetables, extolling the "magical" qualities of vitamin A and vitamin C. Unaware that fruits have almost no protein and few, if any, B vitamins, these fruitaholics, as I call them, deprive themselves of essential nutrients with their one-sided approach to eating. Just like the big meat-eaters, they mistakenly believe that some foods are wonderful while others are terrible.

We search for the perfect way to manipulate our food so we can perform better and feel better. But too often our pursuit of the new upsets what is good about the old.

God didn't give us apple juice or carrot juice or refined rice or white flour. He gave us apples and carrots and whole grains. In the same way that we cut down forests to improve our lifestyle, we hunt for ways to "improve" our diet. We fail to realize that a *variety* of foods — eaten as close to their natural state as possible — is what the liver and the kidneys and the intestines expect to receive.

Put a variety of low-fat, high-fiber foods into your body. Let your organs perform their magic. Isn't it magical the way foods that occur naturally fit so well with our body's needs? What a shame to look so hard for the miracle food when the real miracle is all around you.

PART TWO

Recipes for Smart Eating

14

About the Recipes

WELCOME TO OUR RECIPES! Some people find the rules and principles introduced in Part One easier to apply when they have some recipes to get them started. So we've included here two hundred of our favorites.

Fat Information

Note that for each recipe both the grams of fat per serving and the percentage of fat in the whole recipe are listed. I want you to focus on the grams of fat because the percentage can be misleading, as I explain on page 47.

Food Targets

Each recipe also has a small Target to help you visualize its contribution to a balanced diet. The numbers aren't meant to be super-scientific but rather guidelines. For example, the Target for Jail-house Stew (p. 94) looks like this:

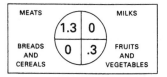

It tells you at a glance that this recipe gives you one and three-tenths servings from the meat group and a three-tenths serving from fruits and vegetables.

The Target for each recipe includes all the listed ingredients except those labeled as optional. Elizabeth Braithwaite, R.D., provided the nutritional analyses, using the Nutritional Database in the *Lifestyles Planner*, a menu-planning and recipe database software program developed by Ronda Gates.*

The next obvious question is: "How big is a serving?" If you're used to a big bowl of cereal each morning, for you that big bowl is a serving. Another person may be used to only a quarter of a bowl, which he assumes is a serving. Our government's new labeling law has standardized serving sizes for packaged foods, and dietitians have provided standard sizes for other foods. For example, three and a half ounces of beef, about the size of a deck of cards, is a serving from the meat group — much smaller than the eight-ounce steak you may be used to having. If I tell you that two servings of meat a day will satisfy your body's needs for iron and niacin, you might eat two eight-ounce steaks to meet that requirement, when all you really need is two three-ounce, low-fat hamburgers or two cups of beans. Here is a quick reference guide for serving sizes.

Meats
One serving =
3 ounces cooked meat
1 cup beans
⅔ cup nuts
4 tablespoons peanut butter
2 eggs

Breads and Cereals
One serving =
1 slice bread
½ English muffin or hamburger roll
⅓ bagel
1 ounce ready-to-eat cereal

---

* The database was created from data in U.S. Department of Agriculture Handbook No. 8, data from manufacturers, and some interpretations of missing values. The percentage of nutrient loss was considered for all cooked foods using U.S. Department of Agriculture Handbook No. 102, *Food Yields Summarized by Different Stages of Preparation.* For comparisons of foods (for example, raw peanuts and popcorn, p. 21), the reference was Pennington and Church, *Food Values of Portions Commonly Used.*

½ cup cooked rice or pasta
3–4 small plain crackers

Milks
One serving =
1 cup milk, yogurt, or frozen yogurt
½ cup cottage cheese
2 ounces cheese

Fruits and Vegetables
One serving =
1 medium apple, banana, or orange
½ cup chopped fruit or vegetable
¾ cup fruit or vegetable juice
1 cup raw leafy vegetable

I urge you to design your food day around the two-two-four-four rule: eat two servings from the meat group, two from milks, four from breads and cereals, and four from fruits and vegetables. Research has established that those minimum amounts will give you (just barely) the adult Recommended Daily Allowance (RDA) for vitamins and minerals. My assumption is that 90 percent of us will eat *more* than the two-two-four-four minimums.

In my clinics, now run by my coauthor, Ronda Gates, we determine realistic weight goals for individuals and then calculate the specific number of servings and grams of fat necessary for them to stay on Target. But for you and me, average Joes who just need to eat sensibly, the miniature Targets with the recipes will keep you on track. If you use several of these recipes on a given day, you can add up the servings from each Target to make sure you meet minimum goals.

Percentage of Fat

With some recipes in the book you'll see an asterisk next to the percentage of fat. That indicates a recipe that may be higher in *percentage* of fat than you would expect from antifat Covert Bailey. There are three reasons for including these recipes.

1. Our intent is to offer smart ways to lower the fat in foods, not to deprive you of good eating. Recipes such as Lemon-Parsley Meat-

balls (p. 100) and Frittata for Four (p. 168), though in the 40 percent fat range, have been modified from the original versions, which are much higher in fat.

2. We don't believe it's necessary to avoid all fat. Some of our recipes have very low-fat ingredients, but we add a dressing to enhance the flavor. A good example is Cucumber-Dill Salad (p. 83), which contains all nonfat, low-calorie ingredients, so when you put the smallest amount of oil dressing on them, the percentage of fat jumps. The recipe may be very low in *grams* of fat even though the percentage of fat seems high.

Look also at the recipe for Grilled Vegetables with Basil Sauce (p. 182). Again the basic ingredients are so low in fat that when you add a little olive oil to prevent the vegetables from sticking to the grill, the percentage of fat seems high. Before you panic about the *percentage* of fat, be sure you check out the *grams*.

3. Our recipes for dips and salad dressings are meant to replace the 100 percent grease dressings people have been using for years. Again the percentage of fat may seem high, but the actual grams of fat and calories per serving are quite low. You can now get fat-free dressings in the supermarket — and I think they're great — but isn't it fun to have that homemade taste now and then?

One last point, and then I hope you'll dive into the recipes. Most of you know how to calculate percentage of fat from the given grams of fat. If you don't, please refer to the box "How to Figure the Percentage of Calories from Fat (p. 49)." With some of our recipes, when you do that you will get a higher or lower percentage than the one listed. The reason is simple: we rounded off the grams of fat in each recipe. Garden Halibut (p. 133), for example, actually has 4.6 grams of fat, which makes the recipe 17 percent fat. When you calculate the percentage using the rounded-off 5 grams of fat, you get 19 percent. We want you to count your total grams of fat each day, but we don't want to make the task harder by giving you decimal points to deal with. So trust us! The percentage of fat in our recipes is correct, even though it may seem a bit off if you calculate it yourself.

This problem with rounding off is particularly evident in recipes containing less than a gram of fat (<1 gram). In a recipe that has less than 1 gram of fat — whether it is .1 gram or .9 gram — the final percentage calculation varies widely. For example, compare the Tuna Spread (p. 55) to the Onion Dip (p. 57). Both have 9 calories per serving and less than 1 gram of fat, yet the onion dip is only 3 percent fat calories while the tuna spread is 15 percent. That's because the actual amount of fat in the Onion Dip is .03 grams, while the amount in the Tuna Spread is .15 grams.

Note also that there's a little bit of fat in almost every food. We think of fruits and vegetables as fat free, but they are not. A half cup of blackberries has .3 grams of fat, and a cup of grapes has .9 grams. An ear of corn has 1 gram of fat, and even a carrot has .1 gram. Knowing this, when you look at some of our fruit and vegetable

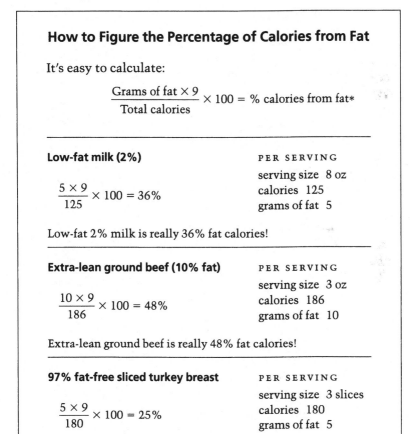

How to Figure the Percentage of Calories from Fat

It's easy to calculate:

$$\frac{\text{Grams of fat} \times 9}{\text{Total calories}} \times 100 = \%\text{ calories from fat*}$$

Low-fat milk (2%)

$$\frac{5 \times 9}{125} \times 100 = 36\%$$

PER SERVING

serving size 8 oz
calories 125
grams of fat 5

Low-fat 2% milk is really 36% fat calories!

Extra-lean ground beef (10% fat)

$$\frac{10 \times 9}{186} \times 100 = 48\%$$

PER SERVING

serving size 3 oz
calories 186
grams of fat 10

Extra-lean ground beef is really 48% fat calories!

97% fat-free sliced turkey breast

$$\frac{5 \times 9}{180} \times 100 = 25\%$$

PER SERVING

serving size 3 slices
calories 180
grams of fat 5

97% fat-free turkey breast is really 25% fat calories!

---

*Calories and grams of fat per serving are listed on most food labels.

recipes you won't be surprised that they have small amounts of fat. The ingredients in the Fruit Flurry (p. 227), for example, seem to be totally devoid of fat, yet it measures 5 percent fat calories. The amount of fat is miniscule — but it's there.

Looking Up the Fats in Food

There are dozens of books for looking up the calories and the grams and percentages of fat in most foods, including packaged foods and fast-food restaurant menus. Among the most popular of these books at our clinics are the following:

Karen Bellerson, *The Complete & Up-To-Date Fat Book*, Avery, 1991.

Jean Carper, *The All-in-One Low Fat Gram Counter*, Bantam, 1980.

Larry Chilnick and others, *The Food Book — The Complete Guide to the Most Popular Brand-Name Foods in the United States*, Dell , 1987.

Michael Jacobson and Sarah Fritschner, *The Fast Food Guide*, Workman, 1991.

15

Appetizers and Snacks

Snacks good enough to serve to guests are five minutes away if you take the time to stock your cupboards with the following foods:

- Packaged hummus mix
  Prepare and serve with wedges of pita bread.
- Nonfat pepper crackers
  Serve with softened nonfat cream cheese.
- Nonfat potato chips or corn chips
  Serve with prepared salsa.
- Water chestnuts or artichoke hearts canned in water
  Drain and serve on toothpicks, dip optional.
- Nonfat bean dip
  Serve with crusty bread or nonfat tortilla chips.
- Frozen grapes or sliced bananas
  Remove from freezer and eat before they thaw.

There's many a night when my craving for snacks is satisfied with a tray of fresh, crisp vegetables, some whole-wheat pita bread, and a low-fat dip. If you just can't give up potato chips, try some of the new nonfat chips. I've had some that actually taste *better* than regular potato chips — and if you combine them with a low-fat dip, you'll never miss the grease.

TANGY CHEESE DIP

Makes 2 cups

1 cup nonfat cottage cheese   4 ounces crumbled blue cheese
1/4 cup nonfat cream cheese

Blend all ingredients together until smooth. Chill for 2 hours to develop flavor.

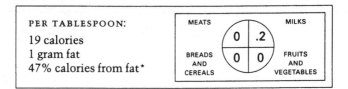

PER TABLESPOON:		
19 calories		
1 gram fat		
47% calories from fat*		

MEATS 0 | .2 MILKS
BREADS AND CEREALS 0 | 0 FRUITS AND VEGETABLES

* See p. 48, no. 3.

EASY RANCH DIP

Makes 1 cup

1 package dry ranch-style   1 tablespoon nonfat
   dressing mix   mayonnaise
1 cup nonfat plain yogurt

Stir together.

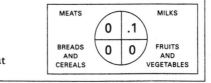

PER TABLESPOON:	MEATS		MILKS
9 calories	0	.1	
<1 gram fat	BREADS AND CEREALS 0	0	FRUITS AND VEGETABLES
3% calories from fat			

SPICY NONFAT BEAN DIP

It's a shame that commercial bean dip changes a nutritious, high-fiber, low-fat food into a lard-filled, artery coating junk food with 60 percent (or more) fat calories. Don't make fun of bean dip. Done right, it's the ultimate health food.

Serves 4

1 16-ounce can pinto beans,   ½ cup picante salsa
   drained and mashed

Place ingredients in a blender and blend until smooth.

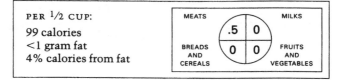

PER ½ CUP:	MEATS		MILKS
99 calories	.5	0	
<1 gram fat	BREADS AND CEREALS 0	0	FRUITS AND VEGETABLES
4% calories from fat			

DILLED VEGETABLE DIP

Makes ¾ cup

½ cup nonfat sour cream
¼ cup nonfat cream cheese
¼ cup chopped green onion

2 teaspoons dried dill
⅛ teaspoon salt
⅛ teaspoon pepper

Combine all ingredients and mix well. Cover and refrigerate 1–2 hours to blend flavors. Stir before serving.

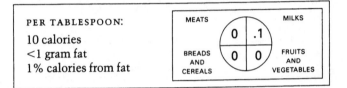

PER TABLESPOON:
10 calories
<1 gram fat
1% calories from fat

MEATS			MILKS
	0	.1	
BREADS AND CEREALS	0	0	FRUITS AND VEGETABLES

SALSA

Makes 4 cups

1 clove garlic, minced
¼ cup chopped parsley
⅓ cup chopped cilantro
1 large onion, chopped
4 large tomatoes, coarsely
  chopped

1 pickled jalapeño pepper,
  finely chopped
1 tablespoon olive oil
2 dashes Tabasco sauce

Mix together all ingredients. Add salt and pepper to taste.

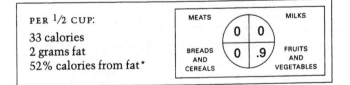

PER ½ CUP:
33 calories
2 grams fat
52% calories from fat*

MEATS			MILKS
	0	0	
BREADS AND CEREALS	0	.9	FRUITS AND VEGETABLES

* See p. 48, no. 2

TUNA SPREAD

Makes 1½ cups

1 6.5-ounce can water-packed
  tuna, drained
½ cup chopped celery
2 tablespoons chopped green
  onion
1 teaspoon dried dill

1 tablespoon lemon juice
2 tablespoons nonfat sour
  cream
2 tablespoons nonfat
  mayonnaise
salt and pepper to taste

Mix all ingredients with a fork until blended. Chill well. If you want a smoother dip, blend in food processor.

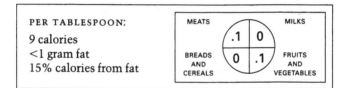

PER TABLESPOON:
9 calories
<1 gram fat
15% calories from fat

	MEATS	MILKS	
	.1	0	
BREADS AND CEREALS	0	.1	FRUITS AND VEGETABLES

TURKEY-HAM SPREAD

Makes 1½ cups

1 cup ground turkey-ham
⅓ cup chopped celery
2 tablespoons pickle relish
½ teaspoon Dijon mustard
½ teaspoon horseradish sauce

3 tablespoons nonfat sour
  cream
2 tablespoons nonfat
  mayonnaise

Mix all ingredients together. Chill well.

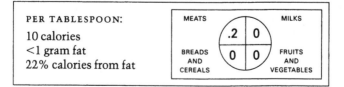

PER TABLESPOON:
10 calories
<1 gram fat
22% calories from fat

	MEATS	MILKS	
	.2	0	
BREADS AND CEREALS	0	0	FRUITS AND VEGETABLES

SALMON BALL

Now that nonfat cream cheese is available, the fat content of this traditional party favorite can be decreased markedly. If you use salmon canned in oil, be sure to rinse it. You can substitute crab or imitation crab for the salmon.

Makes 1 salmon ball

1 6-ounce can salmon
1 8-ounce package nonfat
  cream cheese, softened
1 tablespoon lemon juice
2 tablespoons chopped green
  onion

1 teaspoon horseradish sauce
3 tablespoons chopped fresh
  parsley
salt to taste

Drain and flake salmon, removing skin and bones. Combine with remaining ingredients—except parsley—and mix thoroughly. Chill several hours. Shape salmon mixture into a ball and roll in parsley. Chill well. Serve with low-fat crackers, Melba toast, or thin rye bread.

PER 2 TABLESPOONS:		
33 calories	MEATS .1	MILKS .5
1 gram fat	BREADS AND CEREALS 0	FRUITS AND VEGETABLES 0
23% calories from fat		

One teaspoon of dried herbs is equivalent to three teaspoons of fresh herbs.

QUICHE CUBES

Makes about 30 cubes

¾ cup grated nonfat
   mozzarella cheese
¾ cup grated nonfat cheddar
   cheese
½ teaspoon dried basil

2 ounces diced low-fat
   turkey-ham (labeled 97%
   fat-free)
2 eggs
1 egg white
1 cup nonfat milk

Coat a 1-quart baking dish with nonstick cooking spray. Sprinkle grated cheeses, basil, and turkey-ham into the dish and stir gently to mix.

Beat together eggs, egg white, and milk, and pour over mixture in pan, stirring until well mixed. Bake at 350 degrees for 45 minutes or until quiche is firmly set. Cut into 1-inch cubes. Serve hot or cold.

PER CUBE:	MEATS		MILKS
17 calories		.1	.2
<1 gram fat	BREADS AND CEREALS	0	0	FRUITS AND VEGETABLES
21% calories from fat			

ONION DIP

Makes 1 cup

1 cup nonfat plain yogurt
1 teaspoon onion powder

1 teaspoon lemon juice

Stir together. Add salt to taste. Chill if desired.

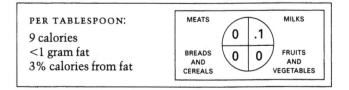

PER TABLESPOON:	MEATS		MILKS
9 calories		0	.1
<1 gram fat	BREADS AND CEREALS	0	0	FRUITS AND VEGETABLES
3% calories from fat			

VEGETABLE CRISPS

Instead of deep-frying your vegetables, try this low-fat technique.

Makes 2 dozen

4 cups raw vegetables cut into ½-inch slices: zucchini, onion, cauliflower, broccoli florets, or any other firm vegetable
1 tablespoon nonfat mayonnaise
2 tablespoons minced green onion
1 tablespoon Dijon mustard or seasoned mustard
¼ teaspoon marjoram and/or thyme
¾ cup soft bread crumbs
½ teaspoon paprika
1 tablespoon melted margarine

Place vegetables on a baking sheet coated with nonstick cooking spray. In a small bowl combine mayonnaise and next three ingredients; stir well. Using a pastry brush, spread ½ teaspoon of mayonnaise mixture over each vegetable. Combine bread crumbs, paprika, and margarine; stir well. Sprinkle evenly over vegetables, turning to coat well. Bake at 450 degrees for 5 minutes or until bread crumbs are browned. Serve warm.

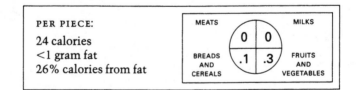

PER PIECE:
24 calories
<1 gram fat
26% calories from fat

MEATS 0   MILKS 0
BREADS AND CEREALS .1   FRUITS AND VEGETABLES .3

*D*on't be too concerned about exact amounts in recipes. For instance, if you really love garlic, use more than the recipe calls for. And if you don't like a particular seasoning, omit or change it. Be adventurous when you cook! Try a recipe with a slight variation each time you prepare it.

16

Soups

LENTIL SOUP

The subtle flavor of chicken broth enhances any dish that calls for water.

Serves 8

4 cups fat-free chicken broth
1 cup dry lentils, rinsed and
   picked over
1 onion, finely chopped
1 celery stalk, finely chopped
1 small green pepper, seeded
   and finely chopped

1 carrot, finely chopped
1 clove garlic, finely chopped
1 small potato, peeled and
   diced
1 cup tomato sauce
½ teaspoon basil

Combine chicken stock, lentils, onion, celery, green pepper, carrot, and garlic and bring to a boil. Reduce heat and simmer about 30 minutes. Add potato and tomato sauce and simmer 15 minutes or until potatoes are tender. Add basil and mix thoroughly.

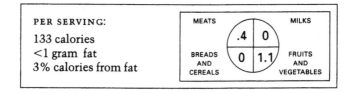

PER SERVING:

133 calories
<1 gram fat
3% calories from fat

MEATS .4 | 0 MILKS
BREADS AND CEREALS 0 | 1.1 FRUITS AND VEGETABLES

SPLIT PEA AND POTATO SOUP

Chunks of potato add taste and texture to this old favorite.

Serves 5

2 teaspoons olive oil
1 medium yellow onion,
  chopped
2 cups beef or chicken broth
2 cups water

2 medium potatoes, peeled and
  quartered
½ cup dried split green peas,
  rinsed
¼ teaspoon black pepper

Heat olive oil over medium heat, add chopped onions, and cook uncovered until soft. Or you can microwave the onions in water and avoid using oil. Stir in the broth and water and bring to a gentle boil. Add potatoes and peas and reduce heat to low, cooking until vegetables are tender, about 40 minutes. Remove from heat and cool for 10 minutes.

Using a food processor or blender, purée the soup in small batches. (Each batch will take about 15 seconds.) Return soup to pot and slowly heat to serving temperature, stirring often. Add black pepper and stir.

Optional: add a dollop of nonfat sour cream or plain nonfat yogurt.

PER SERVING:
137 calories
2 grams fat
15% calories from fat

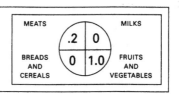

MEATS		MILKS
	.2	0
BREADS AND CEREALS	0	1.0
		FRUITS AND VEGETABLES

VEGETABLE-BEAN SOUP

To speed the preparation of this hearty soup use frozen or canned mixed vegetables (about 8 cups).

Serves 12

1 cup chopped potato
2 cups chopped carrots
2 cups chopped onion
3 quarts water
2 cups fresh green beans
1 cup macaroni
 dash salt
¼ cup tomato paste

3 cloves garlic, mashed
2 tablespoons fresh basil or 2
 teaspoons dry basil
1 teaspoon parsley
¼ cup grated Parmesan cheese
1 16-ounce can white beans,
 drained

Boil potatoes, carrots, and onions in 3 quarts water until almost cooked. Add green beans, macaroni, and salt. Cook until tender. In a separate bowl combine tomato paste, garlic, basil, parsley, and cheese. Slowly add about 2 cups of the hot soup, beating vigorously to blend. Pour mixture back into soup pot, stir, and add beans. Serve hot.

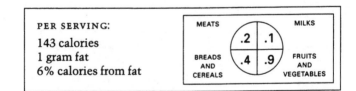

PER SERVING:

143 calories
1 gram fat
6% calories from fat

MEATS   MILKS

.2   .1

BREADS   FRUITS
AND   AND
CEREALS .4   .9   VEGETABLES

Some people are forever going on and off diets. They lose five pounds on one diet, then gain seven when they stop dieting. So they go on another diet, lose more weight, and gain back even more. Their weight goes up and down like a yo-yo. We call it the rhythm method of girth control!

VITAMIN-PACKED MINESTRONE

This soup takes time to prepare, but it's hearty, flavorful, and nutritious.

Serves 8

¾ cup dried navy beans
dash salt
4 whole peppercorns
4 cups (1 28-ounce can) canned
   tomatoes, drained, with
   juice reserved
1 cup chopped celery with
   some leaves

1 cup chopped onion
1 clove garlic, minced
¼ cup chopped parsley
2 cups shredded cabbage
1 zucchini, sliced thin
1 cup elbow macaroni, cooked

Soak navy beans in 8 cups of water overnight. The next day drain water from beans. Place in a large pot and add another 8 cups of water. Bring to a boil, then reduce heat; add salt, peppercorns, and tomatoes (reserving juice). Cover and simmer 1 hour. In a small pan cook celery, onion, and garlic with 2 tablespoons water until tender. Add to bean mixture. Now add parsley and reserved juice from tomatoes. Bring to a boil, reduce heat, and simmer, covered, 1 hour. Add cabbage, zucchini, and macaroni. Simmer until vegetables are just cooked.

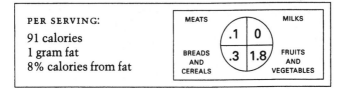

PER SERVING:
91 calories
1 gram fat
8% calories from fat

MEATS .1 | 0 MILKS
BREADS AND CEREALS .3 | 1.8 FRUITS AND VEGETABLES

CHICKEN-BARLEY SOUP

Get in the habit of adding barley to your soups — it's an easy way to increase the fiber in your diet.

Serves 4

4 cups fat-free chicken broth
1/2 cup pearl barley
1/4 teaspoon dried basil
1/2 cup chopped celery

1 cup chopped carrots
1/2 cup chopped onion
1 cup chopped mushrooms

In a large saucepan, simmer broth, barley, basil, celery, carrots, and onion together until barley is tender, about 1 hour. Add mushrooms and simmer 15 minutes. Add salt to taste if desired.

For a heartier soup add 1 cup cooked skinless, boneless chicken breast, diced.

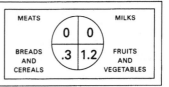

PER SERVING:

83 calories
<1 gram fat
4% calories from fat

MEATS	MILKS
0	0
BREADS AND CEREALS	FRUITS AND VEGETABLES
.3	1.2

TOMATO-LENTIL SOUP

Lentils have all the nutrition of meat but none of the fat.

Serves 10

1 cup lentils
1 teaspoon oil
1 cup chopped onion
1 clove garlic, minced
1/2 cup chopped celery

2 cups chopped tomatoes (fresh or canned)
dash salt
6 cups beef broth
1 large potato, cubed

Place lentils and 3 cups water in large pot, bring to boil, then cover and simmer 1 hour. Do *not* drain. Heat oil in nonstick skillet; add onion, garlic, and celery; simmer 5 minutes. Add vegetable mixture to lentils, along with tomatoes, salt, and beef broth. Simmer 2 hours. Add potato, simmer 30 more minutes. Adjust salt.

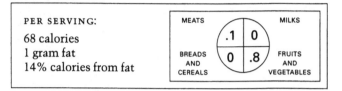

PER SERVING:
68 calories
1 gram fat
14% calories from fat

MEATS   MILKS
.1   0
BREADS   FRUITS
AND   0   .8   AND
CEREALS   VEGETABLES

TARRAGON-BASIL SHRIMP SOUP

Usually used to flavor meat dishes, tarragon and basil give a zesty flavor to the shrimp.

Serves 4

1 cup sliced fresh mushrooms
1 medium zucchini, sliced
  lengthwise in strips
2 tablespoons snipped fresh
  parsley
2½ cups chicken broth
⅓ cup white wine

¼ teaspoon dried tarragon
  leaves
¼ teaspoon dried basil
½ pound small shrimp, shelled
  and deveined
salt and pepper to taste

In a 1½-quart casserole dish, combine mushrooms, zucchini, and parsley. Microwave on high for 3–4 minutes or until zucchini is tender-crisp, stirring once. (Or you can stir-fry the vegetables in a skillet coated with nonstick spray.) Stir in remaining ingredients except shrimp. Microwave on high for 7–9 minutes or until mixture boils. Stir in shrimp. Reduce to medium power and microwave for 3–4 minutes or until shrimp are opaque, stirring once.

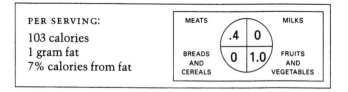

PER SERVING:
103 calories
1 gram fat
7% calories from fat

MEATS   MILKS
.4   0
BREADS   FRUITS
AND   0   1.0 AND
CEREALS   VEGETABLES

HAWAIIAN CHOWDER

Most chowders are loaded with creamy calories. This one is tomato based, low in fat, costs little, and is easy to prepare. We guarantee you'll scrape the bottom of the pot to finish it! Serve with crusty French bread for "dunking."

Serves 10

1 onion, chopped
1 green pepper, chopped
1 clove garlic, minced
1 teaspoon oil
4 cups (1 28-ounce can)
   Cajun-style stewed tomatoes
½ teaspoon dried thyme

2 cups dry white wine
2 cups water
2 tablespoons lemon juice
2 potatoes, peeled and diced
2½ pounds fish (red snapper, tuna, sole)

In a large, heavy-bottomed pot, brown onion, green pepper, and garlic in oil. Add tomatoes, thyme, wine, water, and lemon juice. Bring to a boil; simmer 30 minutes. Add potatoes; cook 15 minutes or until soft. Cut fish in 1-inch cubes, add to soup, and cook 2–3 minutes or just until fish flakes. Serve with French bread.

Caution: It's easy to overcook fish — be ready to eat before you add it to the pot.

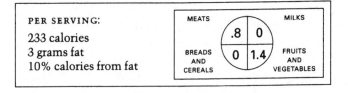

PER SERVING:
233 calories
3 grams fat
10% calories from fat

MEATS .8   MILKS 0
BREADS AND CEREALS 0   FRUITS AND VEGETABLES 1.4

"CREAM" OF ASPARAGUS SOUP

If you used cream in this soup, you'd have 15 grams of fat per serving. By substituting nonfat yogurt, you have only 2 grams of fat — and it's still delicious!

Serves 4

4 cups fat-free chicken broth	*¼ cup chopped onion*
2 cups chopped fresh asparagus	*1 cup nonfat plain yogurt*
(or 1 can)	

Heat chicken broth. Add asparagus and onion and cook until soft. Cool slightly, then, using a food processor or blender, purée the soup in small batches. Pour blended portions into another pot, add yogurt, and reheat gently. Serve at once.

PER SERVING:

72 calories

<1 gram fat

5% calories from fat

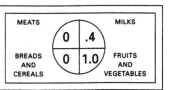

The American public has been dieting for forty years and has GAINED five pounds.

HOT BORSCHT

Borscht is traditionally served with a dollop of sour cream. To keep it fat-free we've substituted nonfat sour cream. Add dark pumpernickel bread for dipping and Russian music to make an ethnic meal.

Serves 6

½ cup chopped onion
1 16-ounce can sliced beets,
    not drained
2 cups shredded cabbage
½ cup chopped carrot

½ cup diced potato
2 tablespoons vinegar
4 cups beef stock
¼ cup nonfat sour cream

Combine all ingredients except sour cream in a large pot and simmer for 1 hour or until vegetables are tender. Cool slightly, then, using a food processor or blender, purée the soup in small batches. Return blended portions to the pot and heat through. Serve in wide bowls with 1 tablespoon of sour cream in the center of each serving.

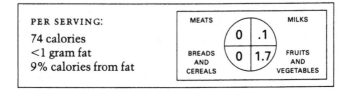

PER SERVING:
74 calories
<1 gram fat
9% calories from fat

	MEATS		MILKS
	0	.1	
BREADS AND CEREALS	0	1.7	FRUITS AND VEGETABLES

*A*mericans are not suffering from lack of vitamins. They ARE suffering from too little exercise and too much fat.

17

Salads and Salad Dressings

Salads

Salad Dressings

Salads are really soups without water. I know that sounds silly, but think about it. Look at all the stuff you put on your plate at a salad bar — if you added water, you'd have minestrone soup. The difference is that with soups we don't add a bunch of grease called dressings.

Salad bars are safe when you "go for the greens." Pack your plate with raw, undressed vegetables such as cauliflower, broccoli, mushrooms, peppers, tomatoes, cucumbers, and sprouts, adding garbanzo or other beans or peas for extra flavor and nutrition. Skip the bacon bits, fried croutons, and seeds. Vinegar-based or lemon juice dressings are the best — avoid the creamy ones. Prepared potato, pasta, vegetable, and fruit salads made with mayonnaise, oil, or whipping cream are too high in fat — better to make your own low-fat salads at home.

Salads

SUMMER CHICKEN SALAD

Grapes in chicken salad? You'll be surprised at how delicious it is!

Serves 6

2 cups cooked chicken, cubed	½ cup nonfat mayonnaise
1 8-ounce can sliced water chestnuts, drained	1 teaspoon curry powder
½ cup diced celery	1 teaspoon soy sauce
½ cup nonfat sour cream	1 teaspoon lemon juice
	½ pound seedless green grapes

Mix together chicken, water chestnuts, and celery. Blend together sour cream, mayonnaise, curry powder, soy sauce, and lemon juice; pour over the chicken mixture. Stir in grapes. Chill several hours.

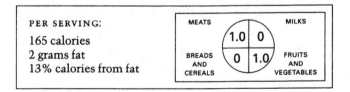

PER SERVING:	MEATS	MILKS
165 calories	1.0	0
2 grams fat	BREADS AND CEREALS	FRUITS AND VEGETABLES
13% calories from fat	0	1.0

CHINESE CHICKEN SALAD

This salad tastes even better if you make it a day ahead.

Serves 2

1 cup cooked boneless, skinless
   chicken, diced
1 8-ounce can water chestnuts,
   drained
½ cup bean sprouts
½ cup chopped celery
¼ cup chopped green onion
2 tablespoons nonfat Italian
   dressing

1 cup cooked brown rice,
   chilled
1 teaspoon soy sauce
1 tablespoon nonfat
   mayonnaise
1 tablespoon nonfat sour cream
1 tablespoon lemon juice

In a large bowl, mix together chicken, water chestnuts, sprouts, celery, and green onion. In a separate bowl, pour Italian dressing over cooked rice and stir until absorbed, then add chicken mixture. In another bowl, mix together soy sauce, mayonnaise, sour cream, and lemon juice, then pour over rice/chicken mixture and toss. Chill well before serving.

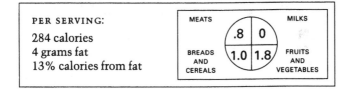

PER SERVING:
284 calories
4 grams fat
13% calories from fat

MEATS .8 | 0 MILKS
BREADS AND CEREALS 1.0 | 1.8 FRUITS AND VEGETABLES

TARRAGON-ORANGE CHICKEN SALAD

Vary the appearance of this salad with colored or unusually shaped pasta.

Serves 4

SALAD

1 cup uncooked bow-tie pasta
  or other small pasta
1½ cups cubed cooked chicken
¾ cup sliced celery

1 11-ounce can mandarin
  orange segments, drained
1 kiwi, peeled and chopped

DRESSING

½ cup nonfat mayonnaise
1 tablespoon grated orange peel
2 teaspoons Dijon mustard

2–3 teaspoons chopped fresh
  tarragon or ½ teaspoon dried

Cook bow-tie pasta according to package directions. Drain; rinse with cold water. In a large bowl, combine salad ingredients except kiwi. In a small bowl, combine all dressing ingredients; blend well. Pour over salad mixture; toss gently to coat. Cover; refrigerate several hours to blend flavors. Just before serving, add kiwi; toss gently.

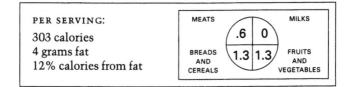

PER SERVING:
303 calories
4 grams fat
12% calories from fat

MEATS .6 | MILKS 0
BREADS AND CEREALS 1.3 | FRUITS AND VEGETABLES 1.3

BLACK BEAN AND CHICKEN SALAD

Black beans give this salad a dramatic color, but garbanzo, pinto, or kidney beans work equally well.

Serves 6

2 16-ounce cans black beans, rinsed and drained
5 stalks celery, finely diced
1 green pepper, finely chopped
2 red onions, 1 chopped and 1 thinly sliced
2 cups cooked boneless chicken breast, diced

½ cup fresh lime or lemon juice
1 tablespoon grated lime or lemon peel
dash hot red pepper sauce
1 teaspoon freshly ground black pepper
red onion rings for garnish

Combine black beans, celery, green pepper, chopped and sliced red onion, and chicken in a large bowl. In a small bowl, combine lime or lemon juice and peel, red pepper sauce, and black pepper. Mix well. Pour dressing over salad and toss well. Salad can be made several hours ahead of time. Garnish with onion rings before serving.

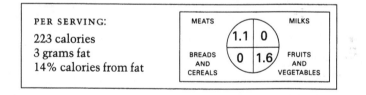

PER SERVING:
223 calories
3 grams fat
14% calories from fat

MEATS 1.1   MILKS 0
BREADS AND CEREALS 0   FRUITS AND VEGETABLES 1.6

BAILEY'S NEW DIET

Here's a radical new diet for you. Stuff yourself, following the four rules of good eating. Eat so many fresh fruits and vegetables, whole-wheat breads, beans, and skim-milk products that you think you'll explode. It sounds crazy, but a lot of people who are successful at weight loss do this.

WILD RICE AND TURKEY SALAD

Try this quick way to use leftover turkey.

Serves 5

1 6-ounce box long grain and wild rice
2 cups frozen small green peas
2 cups cooked diced turkey
1 red pepper, diced

1 Walla Walla or Vidalia onion, diced
1 medium cucumber, chopped
1/2 cup nonfat Italian salad dressing
1/4 cup nonfat sour cream

Cook rice according to package directions, adding peas for last 5 minutes of cooking. Combine rice/pea mixture, turkey, red pepper, onion, and cucumber. Stir in salad dressing and nonfat sour cream. Chill before serving.

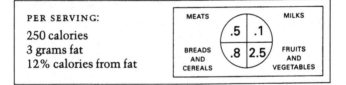

PER SERVING:
250 calories
3 grams fat
12% calories from fat

MEATS .5 | MILKS .1
BREADS AND CEREALS .8 | 2.5 FRUITS AND VEGETABLES

BEANS AND SPROUTS SALAD

Makes 3 1-cup servings

1 8-ounce package frozen green beans, thawed and drained
1 tablespoon chopped green pepper
1 tablespoon sugar
1/8 teaspoon celery seed
1 tablespoon vinegar

1 1/2 teaspoons oil
dash salt and pepper
1/4 cup cubed low-fat Swiss cheese or low-fat cheddar cheese
1/2 cup alfalfa sprouts

In small bowl, combine all ingredients except cheese and alfalfa sprouts; toss gently. Cover; refrigerate at least 2 hours to blend flavors. Just before serving, add cheese and sprouts; toss gently.

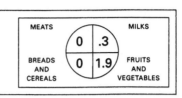

PER SERVING:
96 calories
4 grams fat
39% calories from fat*

MEATS 0 | .3 MILKS
BREADS AND CEREALS 0 | 1.9 FRUITS AND VEGETABLES

THREE-BEAN SALAD

It's fun to vary this recipe by using other combinations of vegetables.

Makes 8 cups

1 16-ounce can cut green beans
1 16-ounce can wax beans
1 16-ounce can garbanzo beans
1 8-ounce can sliced water
  chestnuts

4 carrots, thinly sliced in
  3-inch-long strips
½ cup sliced green onion
1 cup plain nonfat yogurt
1 teaspoon dried dill

Drain beans and water chestnuts. Mix with carrots and onions and stir gently. In a separate bowl mix nonfat yogurt and dill. Let stand 3 minutes, then mix with beans. This can be served immediately, but the salad has more "bite" if it's chilled well first.

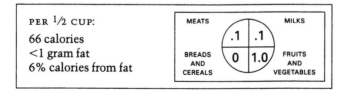

PER ½ CUP:
66 calories
<1 gram fat
6% calories from fat

MEATS .1 | .1 MILKS
BREADS AND CEREALS 0 | 1.0 FRUITS AND VEGETABLES

---

* See p. 48, no. 2.

MEXICALI MIXED BEAN SALAD

Prefer a less spicy salad? Substitute parsley flakes for the cilantro.

Serves 6

SALAD

1 15-ounce can butter beans, rinsed and drained

1 15-ounce can spicy chili beans, undrained

1 15-ounce can kidney beans, rinsed and drained

½ cup sliced celery

½ cup chopped onion

DRESSING

½ cup red wine vinegar

⅓ cup canola oil or vegetable oil

1 tablespoon chopped fresh cilantro or 1 teaspoon dried

½ teaspoon cumin

⅛ teaspoon crushed red pepper flakes (optional)

1 garlic clove, crushed

In large bowl, combine all salad ingredients; mix well. In small jar with tight-fitting lid, combine all dressing ingredients; shake well. Pour over salad mixture; mix gently. Cover and refrigerate at least 1 hour before serving.

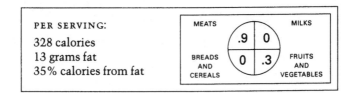

PER SERVING:
328 calories
13 grams fat
35% calories from fat

	MEATS		MILKS
		.9	0
	BREADS AND CEREALS	0	.3
			FRUITS AND VEGETABLES

FRENCH POTATO SALAD

For extra texture (without any extra fat) add chopped cooked egg whites to this salad.

Serves 6

6 medium red potatoes,
 unpeeled (about 2 pounds)
¼ cup chopped green onion
1 2-ounce jar diced pimiento,
 drained
⅓ cup nonfat mayonnaise
2 tablespoons prepared
 mustard

1 tablespoon sugar
2 teaspoons white wine vinegar
dash salt
½ teaspoon celery seed
½ teaspoon pepper
¼ teaspoon garlic powder
¼ teaspoon dried dill

Place potatoes in a medium-sized saucepan; cover with water and bring to a boil. Cover and simmer 25 minutes or until tender. Drain and let cool. Peel potatoes and cut into ½-inch cubes. Combine potatoes, green onion, and pimiento in a medium-sized bowl. In a small bowl, combine mayonnaise and next eight ingredients; stir well. Add to potato mixture; toss gently to coat. Cover and chill.

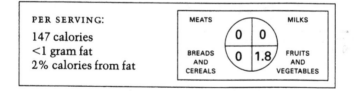

PER SERVING:
147 calories
<1 gram fat
2% calories from fat

MEATS 0   MILKS 0
BREADS AND CEREALS 0   FRUITS AND VEGETABLES 1.8

NEW POTATO SALAD

You can shorten the preparation time of this recipe by using canned potatoes. Be sure to drain the liquid.

Serves 6

2 pounds new potatoes
¼ cup chopped fresh chives
1 clove garlic, minced

1 tablespoon fresh tarragon
¼ cup red wine vinegar
¼ cup nonfat mayonnaise

Place potatoes in a saucepan, add cold water to cover, bring to a boil, and cook until tender, about 25 minutes. Remove from heat and drain. Cool and cut into ¼-inch slices. Place potatoes in a mixing bowl; add chives, garlic, tarragon, vinegar, and mayonnaise. Toss well. Chill before serving.

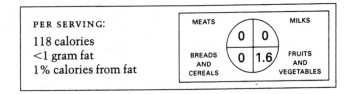

PER SERVING:
118 calories
<1 gram fat
1% calories from fat

MEATS 0   MILKS 0
BREADS AND CEREALS 0   FRUITS AND VEGETABLES 1.6

RICE AND SUMMER SQUASH SALAD

Leftovers from an earlier meal were the basis for this creation.

Serves 4

1 cup cold cooked brown rice	dash salt
¾ cup diced cooked yellow summer squash	¼ cup Italian Herb Dressing (see p. 86) or a low-calorie zesty Italian dressing
¾ cup diced seeded cucumber	
¼ cup chopped red onion	

In medium bowl, combine all ingredients except dressing; mix well. Just before serving, pour dressing over salad; stir to mix.

PER SERVING:

43 calories
<1 gram fat
6% calories from fat

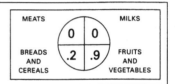

COUSCOUS-SPINACH-TOMATO SALAD

Serves 4

SALAD

¾ cup chicken broth	¼ cup chopped onion
½ cup uncooked couscous	1 cup chopped Italian plum tomatoes
2 cups torn fresh spinach	

DRESSING

1 tablespoon white wine vinegar	1 tablespoon chopped fresh basil or 1 teaspoon dried
2 teaspoons oil	salt and pepper to taste
1 tablespoon crumbled blue cheese	

Bring chicken broth to a boil in medium saucepan; remove from heat and stir in couscous. Cover and let stand until cool. Meanwhile, in a small bowl, combine all dressing ingredients; blend well.

In large bowl, combine cooled couscous and remaining salad ingredients; mix well. Pour dressing on salad mixture; mix well. Cover; refrigerate approximately 1 hour or until chilled.

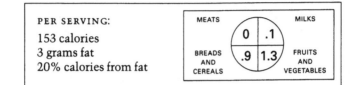

PER SERVING:
153 calories
3 grams fat
20% calories from fat

MEATS 0 | MILKS .1
BREADS AND CEREALS .9 | 1.3 FRUITS AND VEGETABLES

DILLED TOMATOES

Tomatoes have the vitamin A content of vegetables, plus the vitamin C content of fruits.

Serves 6

½ cup nonfat plain yogurt
1 tablespoon nonfat
   mayonnaise
¼ teaspoon dried dill
1½ teaspoons lemon juice

⅛ teaspoon dry mustard
dash cayenne pepper
dash seasoned salt
3 large tomatoes, sliced

In a small bowl, stir yogurt until creamy; stir in mayonnaise, dill, lemon juice, dry mustard, cayenne pepper, and salt. Refrigerate about 1 hour. Place tomatoes in a shallow bowl. Pour dressing over tomatoes.

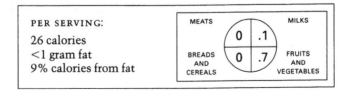

PER SERVING:
26 calories
<1 gram fat
9% calories from fat

MEATS 0 | MILKS .1
BREADS AND CEREALS 0 | .7 FRUITS AND VEGETABLES

SWEET SLAW

Pineapple in cole slaw? You bet. It adds a sweet fresh flavor to the cabbage.

Serves 5

3 cups shredded cabbage
1 4-ounce can crushed
   pineapple, drained
2 carrots, shredded
1 cup nonfat plain yogurt

2 tablespoons sugar
¼ teaspoon celery seed
1 tablespoon vinegar
dash salt

In a large bowl, combine cabbage, pineapple, and shredded carrots. In a small bowl, stir yogurt until creamy. Add remaining ingredients and blend well. Stir yogurt into cabbage mixture.

PER SERVING:
68 calories
<1 gram fat
3% calories from fat

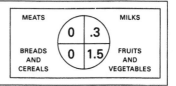

HERBED COTTAGE CHEESE

Serves 6

3 cups low-fat (1%) cottage
  cheese
¾ cup finely chopped green
  onion
1 cup finely diced cucumber

1 tablespoon chopped fresh
  basil
lemon juice to taste
salt and pepper to taste

Place cottage cheese in mixing bowl. Add remaining ingredients
and blend well.

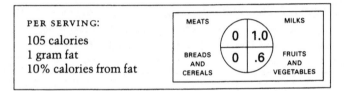

PER SERVING:
105 calories
1 gram fat
10% calories from fat

MEATS 0 | MILKS 1.0
BREADS AND CEREALS 0 | FRUITS AND VEGETABLES .6

CARAWAY COTTAGE CHEESE

The blended spices generate a distinctive, satisfying flavor.

Serves 4

1 16-ounce carton nonfat
  cottage cheese

1 teaspoon Beau Monde
  seasoning (Spice Islands)
¼ teaspoon caraway seed

Combine ingredients. Chill in refrigerator about 20 minutes before
serving.

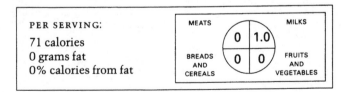

PER SERVING:
71 calories
0 grams fat
0% calories from fat

MEATS 0 | MILKS 1.0
BREADS AND CEREALS 0 | FRUITS AND VEGETABLES 0

*O*verheard at Huckster's Convention: "Every fat person I see eats cottage cheese — so it must be fattening!"

CUCUMBER-DILL SALAD

This is a perfect accompaniment to grilled beef or poultry.

Serves 4

2 cucumbers, peeled and thinly
  sliced
3 tablespoons chopped fresh
  parsley
3 tablespoons chopped fresh
  dill

1½ cups nonfat plain yogurt
2–3 teaspoons fresh lemon juice
1 tablespoon olive oil
3 large cloves garlic, minced
1 teaspoon ground pepper
¾ teaspoon seasoned salt

Toss all ingredients and chill thoroughly.

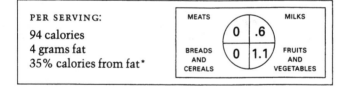

PER SERVING:

94 calories
4 grams fat
35% calories from fat*

	MEATS	MILKS
	0	.6
	0	1.1
BREADS AND CEREALS		FRUITS AND VEGETABLES

* See p. 48, no. 2.

Dressings

Salad dressings are used in such small quantities and thus contribute so few nutrients that they don't warrant the use of Targets.

CREAMY SALAD DRESSING

Our kitchen cupboards contain a medley of flavored vinegars — red wine, tarragon, balsamic, garlic. All of them work well in this salad dressing.

Makes 4 cups

½ envelope unflavored gelatin
¼ cup boiling water
2½ cups nonfat plain yogurt
⅓ cup frozen apple juice
  concentrate
¼ cup balsamic vinegar
¼ cup Parmesan cheese

2 tablespoons olive oil
¼ cup juice from canned beets
  (optional)
3 tablespoons dried onion
  flakes
1 tablespoon Italian seasoning
½ teaspoon garlic powder

Soften gelatin in one tablespoon of cold water; add boiling water to dissolve. Put gelatin and all other ingredients in a blender and mix until smooth. Chill; stir before using. Store in refrigerator.

PER TABLESPOON:

20 calories
<1 gram fat
33% calories from fat*

*M*ost commercial salad dressings are at least 90 percent fat.

* See p. 48, no. 3

RANCH YOGURT DRESSING OR DIP

Few calories! Low fat! Great taste! Who could ask for anything more?

Makes 2 cups

2 cups nonfat plain yogurt
2 teaspoons balsamic vinegar
2 tablespoons powdered nonfat
    milk
1½ teaspoons dried dill
1¼ teaspoons onion powder

1 teaspoon garlic powder
1 teaspoon dried chives
¼ teaspoon dried basil
pinch ground white pepper
salt to taste

Mix all ingredients thoroughly. For best results, prepare one day ahead. Store in refrigerator.

> PER TABLESPOON:
> 10 calories
> <1 gram fat
> 3% calories from fat

DILL-HONEY-MUSTARD DRESSING

Makes 1 cup

1 cup nonfat plain yogurt
1 tablespoon honey mustard

½ teaspoon dried dill
dash hot sauce

Combine ingredients in a bowl and mix well. This is especially good on shrimp salad.

> PER TABLESPOON:
> 10 calories
> <1 gram fat
> 2% calories from fat

ITALIAN HERB DRESSING

This also makes a great marinade for grilled chicken.

Makes 1 cup

¾ cup white grape juice or
   apple juice
¼ cup white wine vinegar
7 teaspoons powdered pectin
1 teaspoon Dijon mustard
2 garlic cloves, crushed

1 teaspoon dried onion flakes
½ teaspoon dried basil
½ teaspoon dried oregano
¼ teaspoon coarsely ground
   black pepper

In small saucepan, combine grape juice, vinegar, pectin, mustard, and garlic; mix well. Bring to a boil; reduce heat to medium. Cook 5 minutes or until slightly thickened, stirring occasionally. Stir in remaining ingredients; blend well. Store in refrigerator. Serve cold.

PER TABLESPOON:

15 calories
<1 gram fat
2% calories from fat

ZESTY AVOCADO DRESSING

This dressing can also be used as a low-fat guacamole dip or as a topping for Mexican dishes.

Makes 2 cups

1 ripe avocado, peeled and
    pitted
⅔ cup nonfat buttermilk
⅓ cup low-fat cottage cheese
1 teaspoon Worcestershire
    sauce

1 clove garlic, pressed or
    crushed
dash salt
dash cayenne pepper

Put all ingredients in a blender and blend until smooth. Thicken, if desired, with nonfat cream cheese.

> PER TABLESPOON:
> 14 calories
> 1 g fat
> 66% calories from fat

If you don't have buttermilk, you can add 2 tablespoons of lemon juice or vinegar to ⅔ cup of nonfat milk for the same result. Or you can substitute an equal quantity of plain non-fat yogurt.

18

Meat Dishes

I have to laugh when those "holier-than-thou" people say, "I don't eat red meat." What do they eat — green meat? Beef is one of the best sources of iron and high-quality protein. Just learn which cuts are lower in fat. Round steak is only about 20 percent fat calories. Compare that to salmon at 40 percent fat calories! Instead of saying, "I don't eat red meat," wise up! Tell people, "I don't eat *greasy* meat!"

HERB-MARINATED ROAST BEEF

You can substitute lamb, veal, or venison for the beef.

Serves 8

½ cup red wine or beef broth
¼ cup oil
1 tablespoon chopped fresh
  thyme
1 tablespoon chopped fresh
  parsley

1 tablespoon chopped fresh
  rosemary
2 garlic cloves, crushed
½ teaspoon salt
¼ teaspoon pepper
2 pounds top round beef roast

In a small bowl combine first eight ingredients; blend well. Remove any visible fat from roast, place in nonmetal bowl or plastic bag and pour marinade over it. Cover bowl or seal bag and refrigerate. Marinate 8–10 hours, turning roast several times.

Heat oven to 350 degrees. Drain roast, reserving marinade. Place roast on rack in shallow roasting pan. Insert meat thermometer. Roast uncovered, basting occasionally with marinade, until meat thermometer registers 160 degrees F (medium doneness), about 1½ to 2½ hours. Let stand 10 minutes before slicing.

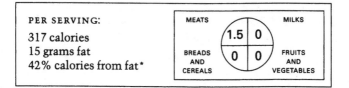

PER SERVING:	MEATS		MILKS
317 calories		1.5 | 0	
15 grams fat	BREADS AND CEREALS	0 | 0	FRUITS AND VEGETABLES
42% calories from fat*			

* See p. 47, no. 1.

MARINADES

Low-fat cuts of meat are often less tender and tasty than the fattier cuts. Marinades are a great way to counter the problem. A good marinade adds spicy or pungent flavors and tantalizing smells to meats, fish, game, poultry, and vegetables. Some are light, consisting of lemon juice or vinegar mixed with a little oil and spices, while others, such as bottled salad dressings or barbecue or steak sauce, are heartier. The sauce section of your supermarket is filled with products that make great marinades. Check the fat content before buying.

PEPE'S PEPPER STEAK

If you are looking for a low-fat cut of beef, use flank steak.

Serves 6

1 pound flank steak
1 cup chopped onions
1 cup defatted beef broth
1 tablespoon low-sodium soy
  sauce
1 clove garlic, minced

2 green peppers, sliced
2 tablespoons cornstarch
¼ cup cold water
2 teaspoons chili powder
2 tomatoes, peeled and cut
  into eighths

Trim fat from meat and cut into 6 serving pieces. Place in a non-stick skillet and brown on both sides. Push meat to one side. Add onion; cook and stir until tender. Stir in broth, soy sauce, and garlic. Cover and simmer 10 minutes or until meat is tender. Add green peppers; cover and simmer 5 minutes. Mix cornstarch and water; stir gradually into meat mixture. Cook, stirring constantly, until mixture thickens and boils. Boil and stir 1 minute. Add chili powder and tomatoes; heat thoroughly. Serve over brown rice or noodles.

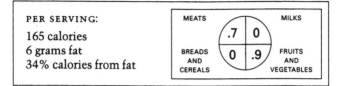

PER SERVING:	MEATS		MILKS
165 calories		.7 | 0	
6 grams fat	BREADS AND CEREALS	0 | .9	FRUITS AND VEGETABLES
34% calories from fat			

STIR-FRY BEEF AND VEGETABLES

Although it takes longer, you can stir-fry the rice before adding the water to give it a crisper texture.

Serves 4

¾ pound boneless top round steak
2 tablespoons teriyaki sauce
1 tablespoon water
2 teaspoons sugar
1½ teaspoons cornstarch

1 cup snow peas
¼ pound mushrooms, sliced
3 green onions, sliced
1 clove garlic, minced
2 cups cooked brown rice

Partially freeze the beef, then bias-slice it into thin strips. Combine teriyaki sauce, water, sugar, and cornstarch. Spray skillet or wok with nonstick cooking spray; preheat over high heat. Add snow peas, mushrooms, green onions, and garlic; cook and stir 2–3 minutes or until tender; remove from skillet. Stir-fry beef until tender; push away from center of skillet. Add teriyaki sauce mixture; cook and stir until sauce is bubbly. Stir in vegetable mixture and mix until heated through; serve over brown rice.

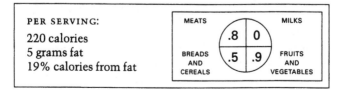

PER SERVING:	MEATS		MILKS
220 calories		.8 | 0	
5 grams fat	BREADS AND CEREALS	.5 | .9	FRUITS AND VEGETABLES
19% calories from fat			

Yes, beef tends to be high in fat. But instead of cutting it out of your diet completely (and, thereby cutting out an excellent source of high-quality protein and iron), learn to use it as the Chinese do. They cook with lots of vegetables and add small amounts of meat for flavor.

DILLY TOMATO-BEEF STEW

If you serve this over noodles or rice, it will stretch to feed eight (and have 4.5 grams of fat per serving).

Serves 4

1 pound lean sirloin
1 teaspoon oil
½ cup chopped onion
2 cups stewed tomatoes,
    undrained
½ cup white wine or water

½ teaspoon dried dill
dash salt
1 tablespoon cornstarch
1 tablespoon water
¼ cup nonfat plain yogurt
    (optional)

Cut sirloin into 1-inch cubes. Brown in hot nonstick skillet, then transfer to saucepan. Heat oil in skillet, add onion, and cook for 3 minutes. Add tomatoes, wine, dill, and salt to onion, bring to a boil, then pour mixture over sirloin and simmer 1 ½ hours or until meat is tender.

Mix cornstarch and water together and add to sauce; bring sauce to a boil and cook until thick. For those who love the taste of Stroganoff, add yogurt and cook gently until heated through.

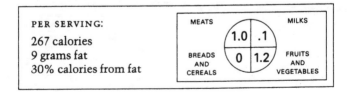

PER SERVING:
267 calories
9 grams fat
30% calories from fat

	MEATS	MILKS
	1.0	.1
BREADS AND CEREALS	0	1.2	FRUITS AND VEGETABLES

IRISH STEW

The longer you cook this, the better it tastes.

Serves 8

*2 pounds lean beef, cut into
  bite-size chunks
1 bottle dark beer
1 pound baby carrots
1 pound pearl onions, peeled
5 cups small red new potatoes,
  whole*

*2 cups beef bouillon
4 cloves garlic, minced
salt and pepper
1 tablespoon cornstarch
⅓ cup water*

Spray a large nonstick Dutch oven with nonstick cooking spray. Lightly brown beef (it will create its own juice); add beer, vegetables, and beef bouillon. Cover and bring to a boil, reduce heat, and simmer 40 minutes. Add garlic and salt and pepper to taste; continue to simmer another hour. Combine cornstarch and water and blend well; stir into the stew and simmer another 30 minutes.

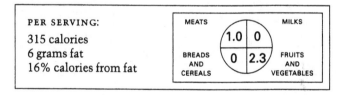

PER SERVING:
315 calories
6 grams fat
16% calories from fat

MEATS 1.0   MILKS 0
BREADS AND CEREALS 0   FRUITS AND VEGETABLES 2.3

*A*n easy way to skim the fat off a cooked dish is to dip an ice cube into the fat. The fat will congeal, making it easy to scoop away.

JAILHOUSE STEW

Here is a dish that takes minutes to prepare, then gives you lots of time to relax while it cooks.

Serves 6

½ pound extra-lean ground beef
1 large onion, diced
⅓ cup brown sugar
½ cup ketchup
2 tablespoons red wine vinegar
1 tablespoon Dijon mustard

1 16-ounce can navy beans, rinsed
1 16-ounce can kidney beans, rinsed
1 16-ounce can butter beans, rinsed

Heat oven to 300 degrees. Brown ground meat and onion in non-stick skillet; drain off any fat. Place in a casserole dish, mix in remaining ingredients, and bake in 300-degree oven for 1½ hours. Cook in slow cooker if desired. Serve hot.

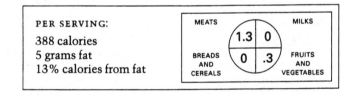

PER SERVING:	MEATS		MILKS
388 calories		1.3	0
5 grams fat	BREADS AND CEREALS	0	.3	FRUITS AND VEGETABLES
13% calories from fat			

NOODLES NAPOLI

Even though it has lots of ingredients, this dish doesn't take any longer to prepare than a traditional lasagna recipe.

Serves 8

1 tablespoon olive oil
1 medium onion, finely chopped
1 clove garlic, minced
1 pound extra-lean ground beef
1 8-ounce can mushrooms, sliced
1 8-ounce can tomato sauce
1 6-ounce can tomato paste
1 teaspoon oregano

1 8-ounce package lasagna noodles
1 10-ounce package frozen spinach, thawed and drained
⅓ cup low-fat ricotta cheese or nonfat cottage cheese
1 egg, slightly beaten
¼ cup grated part-skim or nonfat mozzarella cheese

Place olive oil, onion, and garlic in nonstick pan; sauté until slightly browned. Add ground beef and brown 5 minutes, then add mushrooms, tomato sauce, tomato paste, and oregano; simmer 15 minutes.

Heat oven to 350 degrees. Boil lasagna noodles according to package directions; drain. Combine spinach, ricotta or cottage cheese, and egg.

Pour half the tomato-meat mixture into nonstick casserole; cover with layer of noodles. Spread all the spinach mixture over the noodles, add another layer of noodles, and top with the rest of the tomato-meat mixture. Cover and heat at 350 degrees 30 minutes. Remove cover and sprinkle with mozzarella cheese; put under broiler until top sizzles. Serve immediately.

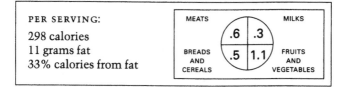

PER SERVING:		
298 calories		
11 grams fat		
33% calories from fat		

MEATS	MILKS
.6	.3
.5	1.1
BREADS AND CEREALS	FRUITS AND VEGETABLES

MEDITERRANEAN MACARONI

This is a good make-ahead casserole. Don't overcook the macaroni — keep it slightly chewy, since it gets additional cooking in the casserole.

Serves 4

½ pound extra-lean ground beef
¼ cup chopped onion
1 cup dry macaroni
½ cup tomato sauce

½ teaspoon dried thyme
¼ teaspoon ground cinnamon
½ teaspoon salt
½ cup grated low-fat cheddar cheese

Heat oven to 375 degrees. Cook macaroni as directed on package. Place ground meat and onion in cold nonstick frying pan and cook until meat is browned; drain any fat. Stir in cooked macaroni, tomato sauce, thyme, cinnamon, and salt.

Spread mixture in an 8-inch-square baking dish. Top with grated cheddar cheese. Bake in 375-degree oven about 35 minutes.

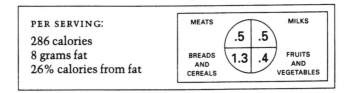

PER SERVING:

286 calories
8 grams fat
26% calories from fat

MEATS .5
MILKS .5
BREADS AND CEREALS 1.3
FRUITS AND VEGETABLES .4

STUFFED ZUCCHINI ITALIANO

Use this recipe in the summer when the garden is overflowing with zucchini.

Serves 4

4 medium zucchini (about 1½ pounds altogether)
½ pound extra-lean ground beef
1 clove garlic, minced
1 teaspoon dried oregano

1 teaspoon dried basil
1 8-ounce can tomato sauce
¾ cup low-fat cottage cheese
2 egg whites
½ cup shredded part-skim mozzarella cheese

Cut each zucchini in half lengthwise; using a grapefruit spoon, scoop out and reserve interior, leaving a ¼-inch shell. Turn shells cut side down in a 12 × 9-inch glass baking dish, cover with wax paper, and microwave 5 minutes or until partially cooked. Let stand covered. Finely chop reserved zucchini pulp. Crumble beef into a 1-quart measuring cup; microwave 3 minutes, stirring once. Drain any fat. Stir garlic, herbs, tomato sauce, and chopped zucchini into beef; microwave, covered, 5 minutes.

Combine cottage cheese and egg whites. Drain excess liquid from zucchini shells. Turn each shell cut side up in baking dish and fill centers with cottage cheese mixture. Spoon meat mixture over zucchini. Cover with wax paper. Microwave 6–10 minutes or until heated through and zucchini shells are tender-crisp. Sprinkle with cheese; microwave, uncovered, 2 minutes or until cheese is melted.

PER SERVING:	MEATS		MILKS
198 calories		.8 | .9	
7 grams fat	BREADS AND CEREALS	0 | 1.1	FRUITS AND VEGETABLES
33% calories from fat			

Here are some smart ways to get the high-quality protein and iron of ground beef while dramatically lowering the fat.

1. *When browning, start with a cold nonstick pan.*
2. *Put a spoon under one edge of the pan and cook the meat on the elevated side to allow the fat to drain off.*
3. *Put the browned meat in a strainer, let it drain, then turn out onto a double layer of paper towels and blot dry.*
4. *For quick defatting, microwave ground beef for two minutes and pour off juices.*

COMPETITION CHILI

For a sweeter flavor, I sometimes add an ounce of semisweet chocolate to this prize-winner.

Serves 6

1 pound top round beef,
  coarsely chopped
1 cup chopped onion
2 cloves garlic, crushed
2 tablespoons chili powder

¹/₄ teaspoon hot pepper sauce
1 tablespoon white vinegar
dash salt
2 cups stewed tomatoes
2 cups canned kidney beans

Brown beef in a deep nonstick pot. Add onion and garlic and cook for 5 minutes. Pour off any accumulated juices and fat. Add all other ingredients. Bring mixture to a boil, then cover and simmer slowly for about 2 hours or until thick.

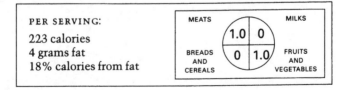

PER SERVING:		MEATS		MILKS
223 calories			1.0	0
4 grams fat		BREADS AND CEREALS	0	1.0	FRUITS AND VEGETABLES
18% calories from fat				

ITALIAN MEAT LOAF

Wow! A meat loaf that includes all four food groups!

Serves 8

1 cup nonfat cracker crumbs,
  crushed
1½ pounds extra-lean ground
  beef
1 6-ounce can tomato paste
2 eggs
1 medium onion, chopped

¼ cup chopped green pepper
⅛ teaspoon pepper
1½ cups nonfat cottage cheese
¼ pound mushrooms, sliced
1 tablespoon fresh parsley
¼ teaspoon dried oregano

Heat oven to 350 degrees. Set aside ½ cup cracker crumbs. In a large mixing bowl, combine remaining crumbs with next eight ingredients; pat half the mixture into bottom of 8-inch-square pan. Combine reserved crumbs with parsley and oregano and spread evenly over meat, then cover with remaining meat mixture. Bake at 350 degrees 1 hour. Let stand before serving. Skim off any fat that floats to the top.

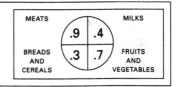

PER SERVING:
267 calories
12 grams fat
40% calories from fat*

MEATS .9 .4 MILKS
BREADS AND CEREALS .3 .7 FRUITS AND VEGETABLES

* See p. 47, no. 1.

LEMON-PARSLEY MEATBALLS

We've added a twist of lemon to traditional meatballs for extra zest.

Serves 4

1 pound extra-lean ground beef	*¼ teaspoon dried thyme*
⅔ cup chopped parsley	*¼ teaspoon grated lemon peel*
½ cup crushed nonfat crackers	*1 tablespoon oil*
1 cup chopped onion	*1½ cups water, divided*
¼ cup nonfat milk	*1 tablespoon lemon juice*
dash salt	*1 tablespoon cornstarch*
¼ teaspoon pepper	*2 cups cooked brown rice*

In large bowl, mix together ground beef, parsley, cracker crumbs, onion, milk, salt, pepper, thyme, and lemon peel. Shape in 1-inch balls and sauté in oil in nonstick skillet. Add 1 cup water. Cover and simmer 10 minutes. Stir together remaining ½ cup water, lemon juice, and cornstarch. Add to skillet, bring to boil, cook and stir 1 minute. Serve meatballs and gravy over rice.

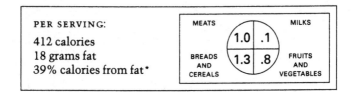

PER SERVING:

412 calories
18 grams fat
39% calories from fat*

MEATS 1.0 | MILKS .1
BREADS AND CEREALS 1.3 | FRUITS AND VEGETABLES .8

* See p. 47, no. 1.

ROSEMARY CRUMB-COATED LAMB CHOPS

This is a great recipe for broiling because the bread crumbs reduce spatter and the cooking spray prevents sticking. There's none of the typical mess caused by broiling.

Serves 4

½ cup dry bread crumbs
¼ cup Dijon mustard
2 teaspoons reduced-calorie margarine, melted
½ teaspoon dried rosemary, crushed

dash salt
¼ teaspoon coarsely ground black pepper
3 garlic cloves, crushed
8 rib lamb chops (about 1 pound)

Lightly spray broiler pan with nonstick cooking spray. Place bread crumbs on waxed paper or in shallow dish. In small bowl, combine mustard, margarine, rosemary, salt, pepper, and garlic; mix well. Lightly spread mustard mixture on all sides of lamb chops; coat with bread crumbs.

Place breaded chops on broiler pan; broil 4–6 inches from heat for 8–10 minutes, turning once, or to desired doneness.

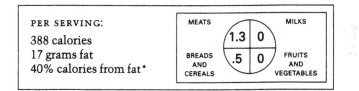

PER SERVING:
388 calories
17 grams fat
40% calories from fat*

MEATS 1.3 MILKS 0
BREADS AND CEREALS .5 FRUITS AND VEGETABLES 0

* See p. 47, no. 1.

LAMB MEDITERRANEAN

Before serving, I add a couple of tablespoons of plain nonfat yogurt to each plate for Milk-group nutrients and Middle Eastern flavor.

Serves 4

1–2 tablespoons olive oil
1 pound lean boneless lamb,
  cut into ½-inch pieces
⅓ cup chopped leek or onion
½ cup chicken broth or white
  wine

1 tablespoon lemon juice
½ teaspoon coriander
¼ teaspoon grated lemon peel
¼ teaspoon pepper
dash salt
2 cups cooked brown rice

Heat oil in large skillet over medium-high heat. Add lamb and leek or onion. Cook until lamb is lightly browned. Stir in chicken broth or white wine, lemon juice, coriander, lemon peel, pepper, and salt. Cover; simmer 20–25 minutes or until lamb is tender.

While lamb is cooking, cook rice as directed on package. Serve lamb and sauce over rice. If desired, garnish with lemon slices and fresh parsley.

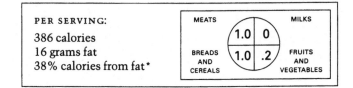

PER SERVING:
386 calories
16 grams fat
38% calories from fat*

MEATS	MILKS
1.0	0
BREADS AND CEREALS 1.0	.2 FRUITS AND VEGETABLES

---

* See p. 47, no. 1.

LEANER SHEPHERD'S PIE

You can substitute extra-lean ground beef for the lamb.

Serves 8

1½ cups chopped onion
2 teaspoons finely chopped
  garlic
½ teaspoon dried thyme
2 pounds ground lamb
1 bay leaf
dash salt and pepper

2 tablespoons flour
1 12-ounce can tomatoes,
  stirred to break up
1–2 pounds small red potatoes
2 cups warm nonfat milk
½ cup low-fat Swiss cheese

In a large nonstick skillet that has been coated with nonstick spray, cook onion and garlic until onion wilts or becomes translucent; sprinkle with thyme. Add ground lamb and bay leaf and allow meat to brown. Drain off any fat. Sprinkle with salt, pepper, and flour. Add tomatoes, stirring constantly. Cover and cook 30 minutes.

Heat oven to 400 degrees. While meat cooks, cut potatoes into 1-inch cubes. Cover with cold water in saucepan, bring to a boil, then simmer until tender, about 20 minutes. Drain potatoes and mash well; add milk and stir until smooth.

Spoon lamb mixture into a 8½ × 14-inch baking dish. Smooth mashed potatoes over meat, then sprinkle with Swiss cheese. Bake at 400 degrees for 20 minutes.

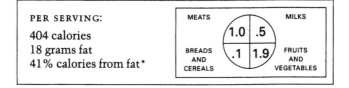

PER SERVING:
404 calories
18 grams fat
41% calories from fat*

MEATS   1.0 | .5   MILKS
BREADS AND CEREALS   .1 | 1.9   FRUITS AND VEGETABLES

* See p. 47, no. 1.

MEDITERRANEAN PITAS

What could you add to these pitas to round out the four food groups? Hint: see page 30.

Serves 8

1 pound lean ground lamb
1 onion, chopped
1 clove garlic, minced
2 cups stewed tomatoes
1½ cups chicken broth
¼ teaspoon dried oregano
dash salt

1 cup brown rice
4 cups chopped fresh spinach
* or lettuce*
4 pitas, cut in half to make 8
* pockets*
¼ cup nonfat sour cream

Place lamb in cold nonstick frying pan and heat slowly until lightly browned on all sides. Add onion and garlic and cook until tender. Stir in tomatoes, broth, oregano, and salt and bring to a boil. Add brown rice, cover, and simmer 45 minutes or until rice is tender. Stir spinach or lettuce into lamb/rice mixture just before serving and heat through.

Meanwhile, in warm oven, heat pita bread until warm. Remove from oven, spread inside with sour cream, and fill with lamb/rice stuffing.

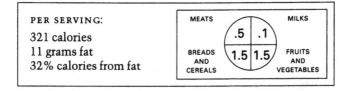

PER SERVING:
321 calories
11 grams fat
32% calories from fat

MEATS .5 | .1 MILKS
BREADS AND CEREALS 1.5 | 1.5 FRUITS AND VEGETABLES

CANADIAN BACON PIZZA

If you bought a frozen Canadian bacon pizza you'd get 41 percent of your calories from fat!

Serves 4

1 12-inch pizza crust or other bread base
1 28-ounce can whole tomatoes, drained and sliced
1 cup shredded low-fat or nonfat cheddar cheese
3 tablespoons prepared fat-free ranch dressing

1 tablespoon prepared barbecue sauce
3 cups finely shredded Romaine lettuce
6 slices low-fat Canadian bacon (Healthy Choice), chopped and heated

Heat oven to 450 degrees. Place pizza crust on nonstick cookie sheet; top with sliced tomatoes; sprinkle with cheese. Bake 8–10 minutes or until crust is crisp and cheese melts. Mix ranch dressing and barbecue sauce in a medium-sized bowl. Add lettuce and Canadian bacon pieces and toss to mix and coat. Spoon on top of hot pizza. Serve immediately.

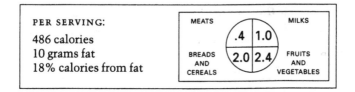

PER SERVING:
486 calories
10 grams fat
18% calories from fat

MEATS .4
MILKS 1.0
BREADS AND CEREALS 2.0
FRUITS AND VEGETABLES 2.4

QUICK QUICHE

I didn't expect a quiche that had a brown-rice crust to taste this good!

Serves 4

1 cup cooked brown rice
2 ounces low-fat ham, diced
2 green onions, chopped
¼ cup cooked mushrooms
½ cup grated low-fat cheddar
   cheese

3 eggs
2 egg whites
1½ cups nonfat milk
dash salt

Heat oven to 350 degrees. Spray 8-inch-square pan with nonstick cooking spray. Press cooked rice into bottom of pan. Sprinkle rice with ham, green onion, mushrooms, and cheese. Beat together eggs, egg whites, milk, and salt and pour into pan. Bake at 350 degrees for about 20 minutes or until quiche is set. Serve hot or cold.

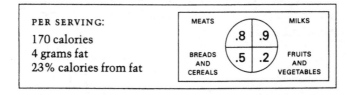

PER SERVING:
170 calories
4 grams fat
23% calories from fat

MEATS .8 MILKS .9
BREADS AND CEREALS .5 FRUITS AND VEGETABLES .2

*A half cup of grated cheddar cheese (2 ounces)
has 18 grams of fat.
A half cup of low-fat cheddar cheese
has 5 grams of fat.*

19

Meatless Main Dishes

MEATLESS CHILI

Red beans, black beans, or pinto beans can be used instead of kidney beans. Or try a combination of all four!

Serves 6

*¼ pound fresh mushrooms,
    sliced*
¾ cup chopped onion
⅓ cup chopped green pepper
1 clove garlic, minced
*1 16-ounce can red kidney
    beans*
*1 14.5-ounce can stewed
    tomatoes*

½ teaspoon ground cumin
½ teaspoon hot sauce
½ teaspoon pepper
¼ teaspoon cayenne pepper
¼ teaspoon dried oregano
*⅓ cup shredded lowfat
    Monterey Jack cheese*
*2 tablespoons sliced green
    onion*

Coat a nonstick pan with nonstick cooking spray and place over medium heat. Heat pan until hot. Add mushrooms, onion, green pepper, and garlic. Sauté for 5 minutes or until vegetables are tender. Stir in next seven ingredients and cook over low heat just until thoroughly heated, stirring occasionally. Sprinkle cheese over top and cook until melted. Garnish with green onions. Serve hot.

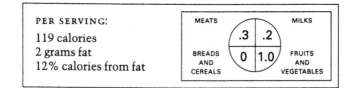

PER SERVING:
119 calories
2 grams fat
12% calories from fat

MEATS .3 | MILKS .2
BREADS AND CEREALS 0 | 1.0 FRUITS AND VEGETABLES

LOW-FAT VEGETARIAN CHILI

Bulgur is a processed form of cracked wheat that provides an excellent base for meatless meals.

Serves 10

1 32-ounce jar tomato juice
1 cup bulgur
1 onion, chopped
2 cloves garlic, chopped
2 teaspoons water
3 carrots, cut into cubes
1 teaspoon ground cumin
1 teaspoon dried basil

1 tablespoon chili powder
dash cayenne
dash salt and pepper
2 15½-ounce cans kidney
  beans, drained
1 28-ounce can tomatoes,
  drained

In a large, heavy saucepan, bring tomato juice to a boil and add bulgur. Cover and cook until bulgur is not crunchy, about 15 minutes. Meanwhile, cook onion and garlic in water in nonstick pan; add carrots and spices, and cook until tender. Add onion-carrot mixture, beans, and canned tomatoes to bulgur. Bring to a boil, then simmer 20–30 minutes. Adjust spices. (You can also use packaged chili seasoning.)

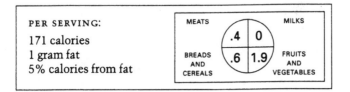

PER SERVING:
171 calories
1 gram fat
5% calories from fat

MEATS   .4   0   MILKS
BREADS
AND   .6   1.9   FRUITS
CEREALS   AND
                 VEGETABLES

*B*eans have the lowest fat of any meat-group food . . . AND they're loaded with calcium, like a milk-group food . . . AND they've got the fiber of breads and cereals. Eat beans — you'll have no friends, but you'll live forever.

MIXED-CAN CHILI

Fast!!

Serves 4

2 14.5-ounce cans Cajun or
   stewed tomatoes
1 10-ounce box frozen corn

1 16-ounce can black beans,
   rinsed and drained

Mix all ingredients in 2-quart saucepan. Heat until bubbly.

PER SERVING:	MEATS		MILKS
224 calories		.5	0
1 gram fat	BREADS AND CEREALS	0	2.5	FRUITS AND VEGETABLES
4% calories from fat			

LENTIL AND RICE CASSEROLE

Double this recipe for a popular potluck dish.

Serves 6

²/₃ cup dried lentils
1 onion, diced
1 clove garlic, minced
5 stalks celery, diced
¼ cup water
1 28-ounce can crushed
   tomatoes

2 cups cooked brown rice
1 teaspoon dried thyme
½ teaspoon salt
¼ teaspoon white pepper
1 teaspoon dried dill
½ cup bread crumbs

Put lentils and 3 cups of water in saucepan and simmer slowly until lentils are tender, about 1 hour. Drain, reserving ½ cup water. Heat oven to 350 degrees. Cook onion, garlic, and celery in ¼ cup water until soft; add tomatoes, lentils, ½ cup lentil cooking water, rice, and spices; mix well and pour into 2-quart nonstick baking pan. Sprinkle with bread crumbs and bake at 350 degrees for 30 minutes.

PER SERVING:			
224 calories			
2 grams fat			
7% calories from fat			

	MEATS	MILKS
	.3	0
	BREADS AND CEREALS 1.0	2.0 FRUITS AND VEGETABLES

BARLEY-LENTIL DISH

I included this recipe because it has pearl barley in it. I'll bet you don't know what it is. I didn't either. I liked it, but I still don't know what pearl barley is.

Serves 2

1 onion, chopped
2 cloves garlic, minced
5–6 large mushrooms, sliced
¼ cup pearl barley
1 teaspoon ground cumin

½ lemon
dash salt and pepper
2 cups nonfat vegetable broth
* or water*
¾ cup lentils

Cook chopped onions in 2–3 tablespoons water; add garlic and mushrooms and stir. Add pearl barley, cumin, juice from ½ lemon, salt, and pepper. Add broth or water and lentils; cover and cook slowly for one hour. (Check regularly, as you may need to add more water.)

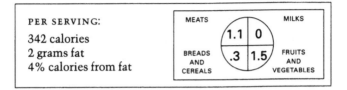

PER SERVING:			
342 calories			
2 grams fat			
4% calories from fat			

	MEATS	MILKS
	1.1	0
	BREADS AND CEREALS .3	1.5 FRUITS AND VEGETABLES

SAVORY BEAN STROGANOFF

This tastes even better the second day, so I often double the recipe.

Serves 6

3 cups chopped mushrooms
2 medium onions, sliced
¼ cup flour
¾ cup vegetable bouillon
4 teaspoons Worcestershire
    sauce
¼ cup sherry or white wine
1 teaspoon garlic powder

½ teaspoon dried marjoram
½ teaspoon dried thyme
¼ teaspoon chili powder
dash nutmeg
3 cups cooked pinto beans
1½ cups nonfat plain yogurt
1 teaspoon fresh-squeezed
    lemon juice

Sauté mushrooms and onions until tender in large nonstick skillet coated with nonstick spray. Mix flour, bouillon, Worcestershire sauce, sherry, garlic powder, marjoram, thyme, chili powder, and nutmeg; add to skillet and cook until thick. Stir in beans and cook over low heat until heated through. Remove from heat and stir in yogurt and lemon juice. Serve over bulgur, rice, or noodles.

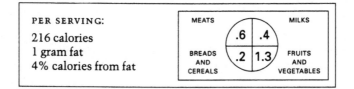

PER SERVING:
216 calories
1 gram fat
4% calories from fat

MEATS .6 | .4 MILKS
BREADS AND CEREALS .2 | 1.3 FRUITS AND VEGETABLES

*W*hole grains, whole fruits, beans, and most vegetables are good sources of dietary fiber, which can help control appetite. When you choose fiber-rich foods, you're eating on Target.

TIJUANA BEAN CASSEROLE

If you add the chili peppers, be sure to tell your guests.

Serves 8

1 cup chopped onion
1 cup chopped celery
1 tablespoon water
1 15-ounce can vegetarian
   refried beans
2 15-ounce cans low-fat
   vegetarian chili with beans

2 10-ounce packages
   whole-kernel frozen corn
½ cup taco sauce
8 corn tortillas, torn up
¼ cup nonfat mozzarella
   cheese, grated
7–8 whole chili peppers
   (optional)

Heat oven to 350 degrees. In saucepan, cook onion and celery in water until tender but not brown, about 3 minutes. Stir in refried beans, chili, corn, and taco sauce. Arrange half the tortilla pieces in a 10 × 9 × 2-inch baking dish; top with half the chili mixture. Repeat these layers. Bake covered in 350-degree oven 45–50 minutes. Sprinkle cheese on top. Bake uncovered 2–3 minutes more to soften cheese. Garnish with whole chili peppers if desired.

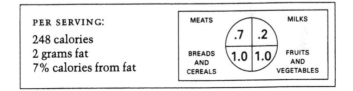

PER SERVING:
248 calories
2 grams fat
7% calories from fat

MEATS .7 | .2 MILKS
BREADS AND CEREALS 1.0 | 1.0 FRUITS AND VEGETABLES

SQUASH AND CHICKPEA PASTA

Chickpeas are sometimes called garbanzo beans.

Serves 6

*1 pound cooked pasta of your
   choice*
1 tablespoon olive oil
*4 medium zucchini or other
   squash, peeled and cut in
   1½-inch chunks*

*1 red or green pepper, cut in
   thin strips*
*1 25-ounce jar fat-free chunky
   garlic and onion tomato
   sauce*
*1 19-ounce can chickpeas,
   drained*

Heat oil in large nonstick skillet. Stir in zucchini and pepper and cook, stirring often, until crisp but tender. Stir in pasta sauce and chickpeas. Heat 2–3 minutes. Stir into cooked pasta, mix well, and serve.

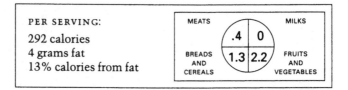

PER SERVING:
292 calories
4 grams fat
13% calories from fat

MEATS .4 | 0 MILKS
BREADS AND CEREALS 1.3 | 2.2 FRUITS AND VEGETABLES

BROCCOLI-STUFFED PASTA

This easy-to-fix dish is a sure winner with dinner guests.

Serves 4

8–10 manicotti noodles

FILLING

1 cup low-fat ricotta cheese
1 cup frozen broccoli florets
*⅓ cup freshly grated Parmesan
   cheese*

¼ cup chopped onion
dash salt
⅛ teaspoon Tabasco sauce

SAUCE

1 16-ounce jar meatless
  spaghetti sauce
1 teaspoon dried basil

2 cloves garlic, crushed
2 tablespoons freshly grated
  Parmesan cheese

Cook manicotti noodles to desired doneness as directed on package. Drain, rinse with hot water, and pat dry.

Heat oven to 350 degrees. In medium bowl, combine all filling ingredients; mix well. Fill each manicotti noodle with 1–2 tablespoons filling mixture. Place in ungreased 12 × 8-inch baking dish.

In small bowl, combine spaghetti sauce, basil and garlic; mix well; spoon over filled noodles; cover baking dish with foil. Bake at 350 degrees 30–40 minutes or until thoroughly heated. Sprinkle with Parmesan cheese; let stand uncovered 2 minutes before serving.

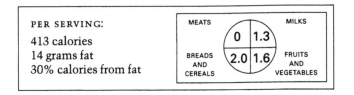

PER SERVING:

413 calories
14 grams fat
30% calories from fat

	MEATS	MILKS	
	0	1.3	
BREADS AND CEREALS	2.0	1.6	FRUITS AND VEGETABLES

*R*ely more on legumes and grains than on meat for daily protein.

SPINACH FETTUCCINE

When I tasted the original of this recipe, I wanted to eat it all! The ingredients, however, included cream cheese, cream, and high-fat cheddar cheese. This low-fat version has the same great taste without the fat calories.

Serves 4

1 12-ounce package fresh
  fettuccine
1 8-ounce package nonfat
  cream cheese
1/4 cup evaporated skim milk
1/2 teaspoon Italian seasoning
1 pint cherry tomatoes, halved

1 10-ounce package frozen
  chopped spinach, thawed
  and squeezed dry
1/2 cup shredded nonfat
  cheddar cheese
1 tablespoon grated Parmesan
  cheese

Cook fettuccine according to package directions. Drain. Meanwhile, in a large saucepan blend cream cheese with milk; add seasoning. Heat cream cheese mixture carefully, and when warm, stir in cherry tomatoes and spinach. Reduce heat, cover and simmer, stirring often, 3–5 minutes or until tomatoes are tender. Add cheeses and stir until melted. Pour over pasta, toss, and serve.

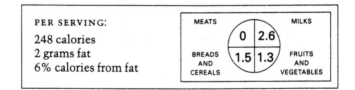

PER SERVING:

248 calories
2 grams fat
6% calories from fat

MEATS	MILKS
0	2.6
BREADS AND CEREALS	FRUITS AND VEGETABLES
1.5	1.3

VEGETABLE LASAGNA

Always cook pasta *al dente* — firm to the bite.

Serves 10

1 pound fresh or 2 cups canned Italian tomatoes, sliced	1 teaspoon olive oil
3 6-ounce cans tomato paste	1 pound zucchini, thinly sliced
1½ tablespoons dried basil	½ pound mushrooms, sliced
1 tablespoon dried oregano	1 pint low-fat cottage cheese
2 cloves garlic, chopped	2 cups part-skim mozzarella cheese
½ cup water	1 cup grated Parmesan cheese
dash salt and pepper	1 8-ounce package lasagna noodles, cooked
½ cup vegetable broth	
1 eggplant, sliced	

Combine tomatoes, tomato paste, 1 tablespoon basil, oregano, garlic, water, salt, and pepper in saucepan and simmer over low heat 20–25 minutes, stirring often to prevent burning. Cook eggplant in nonstick skillet with vegetable broth. Heat olive oil in sauté pan and sauté zucchini, mushrooms, and ½ tablespoon basil until vegetables are softened.

Heat oven to 350 degrees. To assemble the lasagna, spread a small amount of tomato sauce in an 11 x 9-inch casserole; place a layer of noodles on top and spread with more sauce. Put eggplant slices on the sauce, then one third of the cottage cheese, mozzarella, and Parmesan. Repeat layering process with zucchini-mushroom mixture and finish last layer with cheeses. Cover with nonstick-sprayed foil and bake at 350 degrees 1 hour; remove foil and bake at 400 degrees 15–20 minutes.

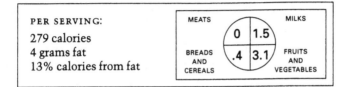

PER SERVING:

279 calories
4 grams fat
13% calories from fat

MEATS   MILKS
0   1.5
BREADS
AND   .4   3.1   FRUITS
AND
CEREALS   VEGETABLES

PAN-BREAD PIZZA

You can use a variety of vegetables in this recipe. For a "classy" pizza use artichokes, and top it with tomato slices.

Serves 4

1 14-ounce flat, round Italian
   bread
1 12-ounce jar meatless pizza
   sauce
½ cup chopped green pepper

⅔ cup chopped onion
1½ cups sliced mushrooms
1 cup grated nonfat mozzarella
   cheese

Heat oven to 425 degrees. Slice unbaked bread in half horizontally and place, cut sides up, on baking sheet. Spread pizza sauce over bread. Top with chopped vegetables and grated cheese. Bake at 425 degrees 15–20 minutes. Remove from oven, cut into wedges, and serve.

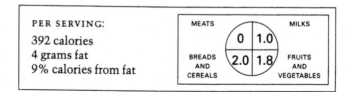

PER SERVING:
392 calories
4 grams fat
9% calories from fat

MEATS 0 | 1.0 MILKS
BREADS AND CEREALS 2.0 | 1.8 FRUITS AND VEGETABLES

People always want to know how many calories they burn during exercise. Rarely do they ask how many calories they burn during the rest of their 23½ hours of daily living. Their half-hour exercise may burn only 300 or 400 calories, while their other activities may burn 2,000. Clearly, most metabolism occurs when we're not exercising. Exercise may not burn a lot of calories while you're doing it, but it influences all the metabolic effects that take place during the rest of the day.

VEGETABLE PIZZA

Compare the fat in this pizza with the 13–17 grams of fat in a serving of sausage pizza!

Serves 8

1 14-ounce pizza crust or other
  flat bread
2 cups shredded low-fat
  mozzarella cheese
2 cups frozen mixed vegetables

¾ teaspoon dried basil or
  Italian seasoning
3 tablespoons grated Parmesan
  cheese

Heat oven to 450 degrees. Place pizza crust on nonstick cookie sheet; sprinkle mozzarella over top, then cover with drained mixed vegetables; sprinkle with basil, then Parmesan cheese. Bake 12–15 minutes or until vegetables are hot and mozzarella bubbles.

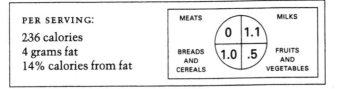

PER SERVING:
236 calories
4 grams fat
14% calories from fat

MEATS · MILKS
0 | 1.1
BREADS AND CEREALS | FRUITS AND VEGETABLES
1.0 | .5

FIBER AND CHOLESTEROL

Not only is fiber good for the colon, it also lowers cholesterol. The body manufactures its own cholesterol from substances in the intestines. Fiber tends to absorb these substances, making them less available for cholesterol production, so less cholesterol ends up in the arteries.

Fiber acts like a drill sergeant. "Okay, let's keep moving! We have to be out of here before sundown. And I don't want any cholesterol malingerers!"

SPINACH-MUSHROOM PIZZA

Isn't it great that the traditional high-fat cheese and sausage pizza is no longer our only choice?

Serves 8

5 cups sliced mushrooms
1 14-ounce pizza crust or other
   flat bread
4 ounces nonfat cream cheese
1 10-ounce box frozen chopped

spinach, thawed, drained,
   and squeezed dry
1 cup shredded nonfat
   mozzarella cheese
3 tablespoons grated Parmesan
   cheese

Heat oven to 350 degrees. Spray large nonstick skillet with nonstick cooking spray; add mushrooms and cook, stirring often, 6–7 minutes or until liquid from mushrooms has cooked off. Place pizza crust on large nonstick cookie sheet; spread with cream cheese, then chopped spinach. Cover with mushrooms, mozzarella, and Parmesan cheese. Bake about 10 minutes.

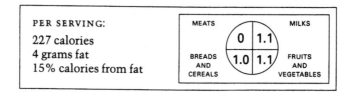

PER SERVING:	MEATS		MILKS
227 calories		0	1.1
4 grams fat	BREADS AND CEREALS	1.0	1.1
15% calories from fat			FRUITS AND VEGETABLES

SPINACH AND MUSHROOM CASSEROLE

This is my version of a spinach salad converted to a casserole.

Serves 6

1 cup nonfat milk
1 cup grated nonfat cheddar
   cheese
1 tablespoon grated onion
dash seasoned salt

1 teaspoon mustard
1 10-ounce package frozen
   chopped spinach, cooked
   and drained
1½ pounds mushrooms, sliced

Heat oven to 350 degrees. Combine milk with grated cheese, onion, salt, and mustard. Line nonstick baking dish or casserole with cooked spinach. Cover with mushrooms and top with milk-cheese mixture. Bake at 350 degrees for 30 minutes.

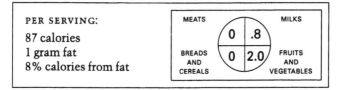

PER SERVING:
87 calories
1 gram fat
8% calories from fat

MEATS 0 | .8 MILKS
BREADS AND CEREALS 0 | 2.0 FRUITS AND VEGETABLES

SPANISH RATATOUILLE

Ratatouille *(ra-ta-TOO-ee)* is a Mediterranean dish. The word means a mixture — of eggplant, squash, and tomatoes. This is a fast microwave version.

Serves 6

¾ pound small new potatoes, cubed
1 medium eggplant, cubed
2 tomatoes, chopped
2 medium zucchini, sliced
1 red or green pepper, sliced
1 onion, thinly sliced
1 6-ounce can spicy tomato juice

2 tablespoons fresh cilantro
2 tablespoons lime juice
1 tablespoon fresh basil
2 tablespoons balsamic vinegar
2 cloves garlic, minced
1½ teaspoons chopped fresh dill

Microwave potatoes in large bowl for 2 minutes then stir in remaining ingredients. Cover. Microwave on high 15 minutes, stirring once or twice to assure that vegetables are well cooked. Remove. Chill and serve.

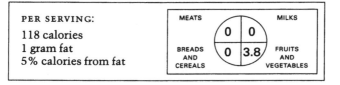

PER SERVING:
118 calories
1 gram fat
5% calories from fat

MEATS 0 | 0 MILKS
BREADS AND CEREALS 0 | 3.8 FRUITS AND VEGETABLES

MARIE'S RATATOUILLE

Don't make the mistake of using a carbon-steel knife to cut egg-plant. I did, and the eggplant turned black. Use stainless steel.

Serves 4

2 cups sliced zucchini	*1 cup seedless purple grapes*
2½ cups diced eggplant	*2 cloves garlic, minced*
1 onion, thinly sliced	*¼ teaspoon pepper*
1 tablespoon vegetable oil	*1½ teaspoons basil*
2 cups diced tomatoes	*fresh lemon juice*

In large nonstick skillet, sauté zucchini, eggplant, and onion in oil until tender. Add remaining ingredients. Lower heat, cover, and cook, stirring occasionally, until grapes are tender. Squirt fresh lemon juice over the dish just before serving.

PER SERVING:

124 calories
4 grams fat
30% calories from fat

	MEATS			MILKS
		0	0	
	BREADS AND CEREALS	0	3.8	FRUITS AND VEGETABLES

CHEESE QUESADILLAS

These are quick and satisfying, especially with a side of beans or rice.

Serves 8

4 ounces shredded nonfat Monterey Jack cheese	*2 teaspoons chopped green chilies*
1 tablespoon chopped fresh cilantro	*4 6-inch flour tortillas*
	2 teaspoons olive oil

Sprinkle shredded cheese, cilantro, and chilies evenly over 2 flour tortillas. Top with remaining tortillas. Brush tops with olive oil. Spray medium-sized nonstick skillet with nonstick cooking spray;

place over medium heat. Heat filled tortillas, one at a time, 2–3 minutes on each side, until tortillas are lightly browned and cheese melts. With spatula, remove quesadillas from skillet to plate. Let stand 5 minutes. Cut each into four wedges.

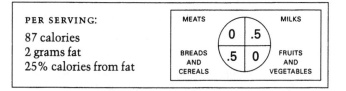

PER SERVING:
87 calories
2 grams fat
25% calories from fat

	MEATS		MILKS
	0	.5	
BREADS AND CEREALS	.5	0	FRUITS AND VEGETABLES

CRUSTLESS QUICHE

You can use chopped spinach, zucchini, or any other vegetable instead of broccoli.

Serves 6

1 10-ounce package frozen
   chopped broccoli
3 eggs
1 cup nonfat plain yogurt
¾ cup evaporated skim milk
2 tablespoons cornstarch

2 cups grated low-fat Swiss
   cheese
1 small onion, chopped
⅓ cup chopped celery
¼ teaspoon nutmeg
pepper to taste

Heat oven to 350 degrees. Cook and drain broccoli according to package directions. Set aside.

Beat together eggs, yogurt, evaporated milk, and cornstarch. Stir in remaining ingredients, except broccoli.

Coat a 9-inch-square baking pan with nonstick cooking spray. Pour egg mixture into pan and arrange broccoli spears on top. Bake at 350 degrees for 30 minutes or until mixture is set.

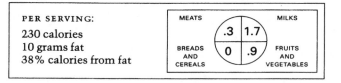

PER SERVING:
230 calories
10 grams fat
38% calories from fat

	MEATS		MILKS
	.3	1.7	
BREADS AND CEREALS	0	.9	FRUITS AND VEGETABLES

COTTAGE CHEESE VEGGIE SANDWICHES

Use English muffins or bagels for a sandwich with more "bite."

Serves 4

1/2 cup shredded low-fat
    cheddar cheese
1/4 cup shredded carrot
1/4 cup chopped green pepper
1/4 cup low-fat cottage cheese

2 tablespoons thinly sliced
    green onion
1/2 teaspoon dried dill
4 slices whole-wheat bread,
    toasted
1/2 cup alfalfa sprouts

In small bowl, combine cheddar cheese, carrot, green pepper, cottage cheese, green onion, and dill; blend well. Spread mixture on each toast slice. Top each with alfalfa sprouts and serve open-faced.

PER SERVING:

103 calories
1 gram fat
10% calories from fat

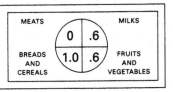

	MEATS	MILKS
BREADS AND CEREALS	0	.6
	1.0	.6
	FRUITS AND VEGETABLES	

*One fast-food double cheeseburger
has 34 grams of fat.*

*Two fast-food grilled chicken-fillet sandwiches
have 16 grams of fat.*

*Four of our cottage cheese veggie sandwiches
have only 4 grams of fat!*

20

Seafood

Sauces

COD WITH GINGER

In New England, cod, a bottom fish, is not as treasured as salmon or halibut. But it's very low in fat, and if you doctor it up using this recipe, you'll have an economical, low-fat — and delicious — dish.

Serves 6

½ cup unsweetened orange juice
2 teaspoons lemon juice
2 teaspoons cornstarch
1 teaspoon low-sodium soy sauce

2 green onions, sliced thin
1½ teaspoons minced fresh ginger
1½ pounds cod fillets
salt and pepper (optional)

Heat oven to 400 degrees. Combine orange juice, lemon juice, cornstarch, and soy sauce in small saucepan. Cook over medium heat until sauce thickens. Stir green onion and ginger into this mixture and remove from heat. Place fish in shallow casserole dish coated with nonstick cooking spray; sprinkle with salt and pepper if desired. Spread sauce over fish and bake at 400 degrees until fish flakes easily with a fork, 8–10 minutes per inch of thickness.

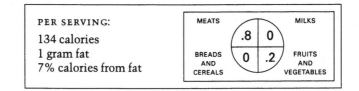

PER SERVING:
134 calories
1 gram fat
7% calories from fat

MEATS .8 | 0 MILKS
BREADS AND CEREALS 0 | .2 FRUITS AND VEGETABLES

CREOLE FISH

Any firm white fish, such as grouper or cod, can be used instead of haddock.

Serves 4

1 pound sole or haddock fillet,
  cut in 4 pieces
1 8-ounce can tomato sauce
1 2-ounce can sliced
  mushrooms, drained
½ cup diced green pepper

1 stalk celery, sliced
1 tablespoon chopped onion
3 tablespoons water
1 teaspoon chicken bouillon
  granules

Rinse fish and pat dry. In a 12 × 8 × 2-inch dish, arrange fish with thickest pieces on the outside. Combine tomato sauce, mushrooms, green pepper, celery, onion, water, and bouillon granules. Pour evenly over fish. Cover tightly with plastic wrap, turning back one corner to vent. Microwave on high 4 minutes, then rotate dish ½ turn. Cook 4–6 minutes or until fish flakes easily with a fork. Let stand about 5 minutes before serving to blend flavors.

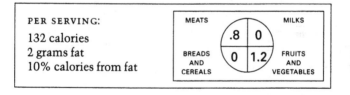

PER SERVING:
132 calories
2 grams fat
10% calories from fat

MEATS   .8   0   MILKS
BREADS AND CEREALS   0   1.2   FRUITS AND VEGETABLES

ORIENTAL HADDOCK

The marinade will keep up to three days. It can also be used as a dressing over a lettuce or spinach salad.

Serves 6

2 tablespoons ketchup
2 tablespoons chopped fresh
*   parsley*
2 teaspoons low-sodium soy
*   sauce*
1½ tablespoons minced fresh
*   ginger*

1 clove garlic, minced
1 tablespoon lemon juice
½ cup orange juice
salt and pepper to taste
1 pound haddock

Mix together all ingredients except fish. Place fish in 9 x 13-inch pan and pour marinade over it. Marinate in refrigerator 1 hour or more, turning fish 2–3 times. Place fish on broiler pan coated with nonstick cooking spray; reserve marinade. Broil fish until it flakes easily with fork, basting once or twice with reserved marinade.

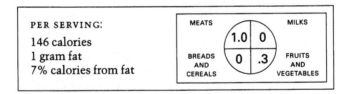

PER SERVING:

146 calories
1 gram fat
7% calories from fat

	MEATS		MILKS
	1.0	0	
BREADS AND CEREALS	0	.3	FRUITS AND VEGETABLES

*T*he lower shelves at your supermarket usually offer better values than shelves at eye level.

POACHED FISH À L'ORANGE

If the sauce is too thick, add more orange juice; if it's too thin, use more cornstarch.

Serves 4

1 cup orange juice
2½ tablespoons sherry
  (optional)
2 teaspoons low-sodium soy
  sauce
dash salt and pepper
1 medium onion, sliced and
  separated into rings
4 medium carrots, sliced thin

1 medium green pepper, cut
  into strips
1 pound skinless fish fillets
  (sole, orange roughy, pike,
  cod)
1 teaspoon cornstarch
¼ cup cold water
1 medium tomato cut into 8
  wedges

In a large nonstick skillet, combine orange juice, sherry, soy sauce, salt, and pepper; add onion and carrots. Bring to a boil; reduce heat and simmer until vegetables are tender-crisp. Stir in green pepper. Push vegetables to edge of skillet. Arrange fish in center of skillet. Bring liquid to a boil; reduce heat. Simmer covered 2–3 minutes, or until fish flakes easily with a fork. Remove fish from skillet. Combine cornstarch and ¼ cup cold water; stir mixture into sauce in skillet. Cook and stir until bubbly, then cook 1–2 minutes more. Return fish to skillet; arrange tomato wedges on top. Serve hot.

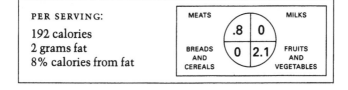

PER SERVING:
192 calories
2 grams fat
8% calories from fat

MEATS   MILKS
.8   0
BREADS AND CEREALS   0   2.1   FRUITS AND VEGETABLES

GRILLED FISH WITH TOMATO-BASIL SAUCE

You can store fresh basil or any other herb by putting the stems in a glass of water in the refrigerator. Change the water daily.

Serves 6

1 pound fish suitable for grilling (halibut, salmon, swordfish, perch)
1 teaspoon olive oil
1 clove garlic, minced
3 large, ripe tomatoes, sliced
1/3 cup chopped onion

1/4 cup lemon juice
1 cup chopped zucchini
dash salt and pepper
1/4 teaspoon sugar
1/4 cup fresh basil or 1 teaspoon dried

Brush fish with olive oil and sprinkle with salt and pepper (optional). Grill on both sides until fish flakes easily with a fork, about 8–10 minutes per inch of thickness. While fish is cooking, cook garlic, tomatoes, onion, lemon juice, and zucchini until vegetables are soft. Add salt, pepper, and sugar. Cook until sauce thickens, 10–13 minutes. Add basil and serve over fish.

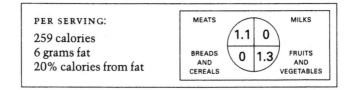

PER SERVING:	MEATS	MILKS
259 calories	1.1	0
6 grams fat	BREADS AND CEREALS	FRUITS AND VEGETABLES
20% calories from fat	0	1.3

If you're fat and you don't exercise, the rule is — eat it today, wear it tomorrow.

CRAB-STUFFED RED SNAPPER

This dish has negligible fat, but the sodium content (about 800 mg per serving) may be too high for some people.
If you have an appropriate-sized pan you can leave the head and tail on the fish for a more dramatic presentation.

Serves 4

1 pound red snapper, cut into 4
*   fillets*
6 ounces cooked crabmeat or
*   imitation crab, finely*
*   chopped*
½ cup shredded carrot
1 green onion, thinly sliced
1 teaspoon sugar

1 teaspoon cornstarch
¼ cup plus 1 teaspoon soy
*   sauce*
¼ cup plus 1 teaspoon dry
*   sherry*
1 tablespoon brown sugar
1 teaspoon grated fresh ginger
1 cup water

Score fish fillets with diagonal cuts on each side, slicing almost through. Combine crabmeat, carrot, green onion, sugar, cornstarch, 1 teaspoon soy sauce, and 1 teaspoon sherry; spoon mixture into fish cavity, patting mixture to flatten evenly. Coat rack of poaching pan with nonstick cooking spray; place fish on rack and lower into poaching pan. Combine ¼ cup soy sauce, ¼ cup sherry, brown sugar, ginger, and water; pour over fish. Simmer, covered, 20 minutes or until fish flakes. Transfer fish to platter, spoon some liquid on top.

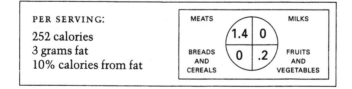

PER SERVING:	MEATS		MILKS
252 calories		1.4	0
3 grams fat	BREADS AND CEREALS	0	.2	FRUITS AND VEGETABLES
10% calories from fat			

STUFFED SOLE

Serve this with French Peas (p. 178).

Serves 4

½ *pound sliced mushrooms*
1 *teaspoon oil*
½ *pound fresh spinach,*
    shredded
¼ *teaspoon garlic powder*
¼ *teaspoon dried oregano*

1½ *pounds sole fillets, in 4*
    pieces
4 *teaspoons lemon juice*
2 *tablespoons grated part-skim*
    mozzarella cheese
paprika

Heat oven to 425 degrees. In large skillet brown mushrooms in oil until limp. Add spinach and cook for one minute. Remove from heat and drain. Add garlic powder and oregano.

Place one quarter of mixture in center of each fillet; roll and place, seam down, in a baking dish coated with nonstick cooking spray. Sprinkle with lemon juice and top with cheese.

Bake in 425-degree oven 20 minutes. Sprinkle a dash of paprika on each roll after removing from oven.

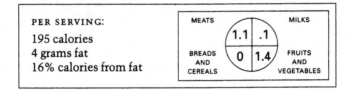

PER SERVING:
195 calories
4 grams fat
16% calories from fat

MEATS 1.1 .1 MILKS
BREADS AND CEREALS 0 1.4 FRUITS AND VEGETABLES

GARDEN HALIBUT

Any white fish is suitable in this recipe.

Serves 6

1 cup chopped carrots	*2 tablespoons white wine*
1 cup chopped celery	*1 teaspoon dried basil*
½ cup sliced onion	*½ teaspoon dried thyme*
½ cup chopped mushrooms	*dash salt and pepper*
1 tablespoon water	*2 pounds halibut steak*

In a nonstick skillet, cook carrots, celery, onion, and mushrooms in water until soft, about 5 minutes. Stir in wine, herbs, salt, and pepper. Simmer covered 1 minute. Place fish on vegetables. Cover and simmer until fish flakes easily with a fork, about 8–10 minutes per inch of thickness.

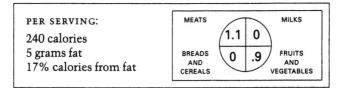

PER SERVING:
240 calories
5 grams fat
17% calories from fat

MEATS 1.1   0 MILKS
BREADS AND CEREALS 0   .9 FRUITS AND VEGETABLES

*D*on't eat extracted *fats. If you want fish oil, eat the fish.* Don't eat Wesson oil, eat the wessons!

SALMON WITH LEMON-ONION COUSCOUS

In most salmon recipes creamy sauces cover the flavor of this deli-
cate Pacific Northwest fish. Try this instead.

Serves 4

*1 tablespoon reduced-calorie
    margarine
½ onion, sliced and separated
    into rings
½ cup defatted chicken broth
¼ cup lemon juice
¼ teaspoon grated lemon peel
    (optional)*

*dash salt and pepper
1 pound salmon, cut into 4
    fillets
½ cup water
½ cup uncooked couscous
4–5 lemon slices (optional)
2 tablespoons chopped fresh
    parsley (optional)*

Melt margarine in large skillet. Add onion rings; cook and stir 1–2
minutes. Stir in chicken broth, lemon juice, lemon peel, salt, and
pepper. Bring to a boil and add salmon. Cover; cook over medium-
high heat 8–9 minutes or until fish flakes easily with fork. Remove
salmon and onion rings from skillet; keep warm. Reserve ¼ cup
of cooking liquid in skillet; discard remaining liquid.

Add water to reserved cooking liquid and bring to a boil. Stir in
couscous. Remove from heat. Cover; let stand 5 minutes. Serve
warm salmon and onion with couscous. Garnish with lemon slices
and parsley.

PER SERVING:		
282 calories	MEATS	MILKS
7 grams fat	.8	0
21% calories from fat	BREADS AND CEREALS .9	.3 FRUITS AND VEGETABLES

LOW-FAT SALMON ROMANOFF

Use fresh whole-wheat pasta to make this dish even higher in fiber.

Serves 4

1 cup nonfat chicken broth
10 ounces fresh salmon
6 ounces pasta, cooked
1 cup nonfat plain yogurt,
    drained

½ package dry ranch-style
    dressing mix
½ cup fresh mushrooms
3 tablespoons chopped green
    onion
¼ teaspoon dried dill

Put chicken broth in skillet and bring to a boil. Add salmon and bring to a second boil. Cover and simmer 4–5 minutes, turn fish over, and cook another 4–5 minutes or until fish flakes easily. Drain off and discard liquid. Break up salmon into bite-size pieces.

    Combine all ingredients, mixing well; place in nonstick, microwave-safe dish. Cook in microwave on medium-high until heated through, about 5 minutes. Stir and serve.

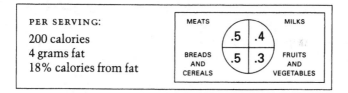

PER SERVING:
200 calories
4 grams fat
18% calories from fat

MEATS .5 .4 MILKS
BREADS AND CEREALS .5 .3 FRUITS AND VEGETABLES

SEAFOOD STIR-FRY

You can use different vegetables, or prepare with chicken or beef — this dish will taste different every time.

Serves 4

¾ pound Pacific snapper, ling,
   or cod fillets
¼ pound raw scallops
⅓ pound tiny cooked shrimp
1½ tablespoons low-sodium
   soy sauce
⅓ cup dry white wine
2 teaspoons cornstarch

¾ cup orange juice
2 tablespoons water
2 teaspoons grated fresh ginger
1 tablespoon minced garlic
2 ounces (1 cup) snow peas
1 red pepper, sliced thin
½ cup sliced green pepper

Rinse fish and shellfish briefly with cold water; drain or pat dry with paper towels. Cut fish into large chunks. Combine soy sauce, wine, cornstarch, and orange juice. Add fish chunks and marinate in refrigerator for 30 minutes. Drain fish and reserve marinade. Heat water in nonstick skillet. Add ginger and garlic and cook 5–10 seconds to release flavors. Add snow peas, red and green pepper, fish chunks, and scallops; stir-fry for 2 minutes. Add shrimp and reserved marinade and cook just until sauce thickens. Serve immediately over rice.

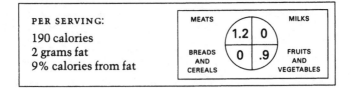

PER SERVING:		
190 calories	MEATS **1.2**	MILKS **0**
2 grams fat	BREADS AND CEREALS **0**	**.9** FRUITS AND VEGETABLES
9% calories from fat		

SHRIMP CREOLE

The bay leaf gives this dish its creole flavor. You can also use creole seasoning.

Serves 6

½ medium onion, chopped
2½ cups water
¼ cup diced celery
1 teaspoon minced parsley
1 green pepper, chopped

1 6-ounce can tomato paste
1 bay leaf, crushed
¼ teaspoon cayenne pepper
2 cups cooked shrimp

In skillet, cook onion in 1 tablespoon water. Blend in all other ingredients except shrimp. Cook slowly, stirring occasionally, about 30 minutes. Stir in shrimp and heat. Serve over rice or noodles.

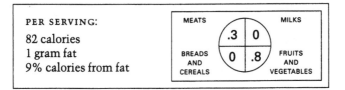

PER SERVING:
82 calories
1 gram fat
9% calories from fat

MEATS .3 / 0 MILKS
BREADS AND CEREALS 0 / .8 FRUITS AND VEGETABLES

*F*at is the most concentrated source of food energy (calories). Each gram of fat supplies about 9 calories, compared with about 4 calories per gram of protein or carbohydrate and 7 calories per gram of alcohol.

MOCK LOBSTER SALAD

Imagine preparing a showcase salad that looks and tastes like lobster but is one quarter the cost. My sister makes this dish for her buffets. I don't think her guests have figured it out yet. Sorry, Barbara — the secret is out!

Serves 6

1 pound halibut (or cod or
   flounder)
1 small onion, sliced
1 bay leaf
¼ teaspoon ground pepper
2 slices lemon
1 tablespoon allspice
dash salt

3 hard-boiled eggs, chopped
1 carrot, grated
1 cup nonfat mayonnaise
½ cup diced celery
½ cup chili sauce
½ cup finely cut strips green
   pepper

Steam halibut with onion, bay leaf, pepper, lemon, allspice, and salt until fish flakes easily (about 12 minutes). While fish is cooking, mix eggs, carrot, mayonnaise, celery, and chili sauce. Break up fish and mix into mayonnaise mixture. Chill thoroughly. Put in a mold and chill several hours before serving. Garnish with green pepper strips.

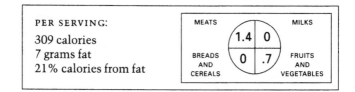

PER SERVING:
309 calories
7 grams fat
21% calories from fat

MEATS 1.4   MILKS 0
BREADS AND CEREALS 0   FRUITS AND VEGETABLES .7

PASTA WITH BROCCOLI AND CLAM SAUCE

If you make this dish with fresh pasta, I suggest steaming the broccoli separately from the pasta.

Serves 4

1 12-ounce package pasta of
   your choice
2 cups broccoli florets

3 tablespoons olive oil
2 cloves garlic, minced
1 6.5-ounce can minced clams

Cook pasta according to package directions, using extra water. About 5 minutes before pasta is done, add broccoli and continue to cook until pasta and broccoli are tender. Drain thoroughly. While pasta is cooking, prepare sauce by heating oil in small saucepan. Add garlic and cook over low heat until tender. Stir in undrained clams, bring to a boil, reduce heat, and simmer 3–5 minutes to develop the flavors. Pour sauce over broccoli-pasta mixture.

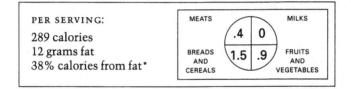

PER SERVING:

289 calories
12 grams fat
38% calories from fat*

MEATS		MILKS
	.4	0
BREADS AND CEREALS	1.5	.9
		FRUITS AND VEGETABLES

*P*asta comes in a variety of shapes, colors, and sizes. Let your children help you decide — Christmas tree shapes for the holidays, heart shapes on Valentine's Day. They'll gobble it up if they've had a say in the selection.

* See p. 48, no. 2

BAKED TUNA SANDWICH

I make this sandwich even wetter by adding lots of tomatoes and shredded lettuce.

Serves 2

1 6.5-ounce can water-packed
  tuna
3 tablespoons nonfat plain
  yogurt
1 tablespoon nonfat
  mayonnaise
½ teaspoon dried dill

2 tablespoons lemon juice
1 tablespoon minced green
  onion
salt and pepper to taste
1 egg white, beaten
2 slices whole-wheat bread

Make a tuna salad with all ingredients except egg white and 1 tablespoon yogurt. Toast bread, and spread tuna on each piece. Mix egg white and 1 tablespoon yogurt together and spread on top of tuna, covering toast completely. Place sandwich under broiler until egg white is cooked and brown, about 1 minute.

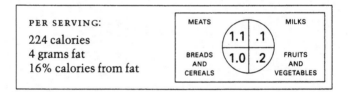

PER SERVING:
224 calories
4 grams fat
16% calories from fat

MEATS 1.1 | .1 MILKS
BREADS AND CEREALS 1.0 | .2 FRUITS AND VEGETABLES

TUNA-BROCCOLI ROLLS

If you're on a budget, this is a good way to serve a large group.

Serves 12

TUNA ROLLS

12 uncooked lasagna noodles
1 10-ounce package frozen
  chopped broccoli, thawed
  and drained

1 6.5-ounce can water-packed
  tuna, drained and flaked
1 4.5-ounce jar sliced
  mushrooms, drained

SAUCE

2 tablespoons reduced-calorie   ½ teaspoon dried thyme
  margarine   salt and pepper to taste
¼ cup flour   ½ cup shredded low-fat
1½ cups nonfat milk   cheddar cheese
1 cup chicken broth

Cook lasagna noodles as directed on package. Drain; rinse with hot water. Meanwhile, in medium bowl, combine broccoli, tuna, and mushrooms; mix well.

Melt margarine in medium saucepan over low heat. Stir in flour to make a paste; gradually add milk and cook, stirring constantly, until mixture is smooth and bubbly. Stir in thyme, salt, and pepper; cook over medium heat 5–8 minutes until sauce is thickened, stirring constantly. Stir half of sauce (1 cup) into broccoli mixture; mix well.

Heat oven to 350 degrees. Spread each cooked lasagna noodle with about 2 heaping tablespoons broccoli mixture. Roll up each noodle; place in ungreased 13 × 9-inch (3-quart) baking dish. Spoon remaining sauce over rolls; cover.

Bake at 350 degrees 25–35 minutes or until thoroughly heated. Remove cover and sprinkle with cheese; bake an additional 5 minutes or until cheese is melted.

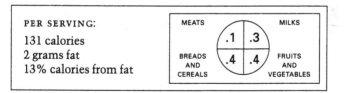

PER SERVING:
131 calories
2 grams fat
13% calories from fat

MEATS .1 | .3 MILKS
BREADS AND CEREALS .4 | .4 FRUITS AND VEGETABLES

TUNA FISH CASSEROLE

This is an easy recipe for kids to make. If you want your children to eat well, let them have a hand in food preparation.

Serves 6

2 6.5-ounce cans water-packed
   tuna, drained
½ cup low-fat cottage cheese

5 white or whole-wheat bread
   slices, cubed

SAUCE

2 tablespoons margarine
3 tablespoons flour
½ cup shredded nonfat
   American cheese

1½ cups nonfat milk
1 teaspoon paprika
salt to taste

Heat oven to 350 degrees. Mix tuna fish with cottage cheese and half the bread cubes; spread in 11 × 7-inch pan. Make sauce by melting margarine in saucepan; add flour and stir. Add cheese and milk and stir until heated and somewhat thick; pour over tuna mixture. Toss remaining bread cubes with paprika and salt. Sprinkle over top. Bake at 350 degrees for 25 minutes.

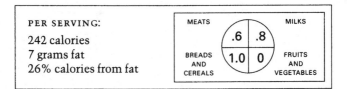

PER SERVING:
242 calories
7 grams fat
26% calories from fat

MEATS: .6
MILKS: .8
BREADS AND CEREALS: 1.0
FRUITS AND VEGETABLES: 0

One 6-ounce can of oil-packed tuna contains
474 calories, 20 grams fat, and 37.2 grams protein.

One 6-ounce can of water-packed tuna contains
186 calories, 1.2 grams fat, and 37.2 grams protein.

DILL SAUCE

This sauce is lower in fat than a typical dill sauce. It is delicious on fish and can double as a salad dressing.

Makes 1/2 cup

1/2 cup nonfat plain yogurt
1 tablespoon vegetable oil
1 tablespoon vinegar

1 tablespoon minced onion
1 tablespoon minced parsley
1/2 teaspoon dried dill

In bowl, stir yogurt until creamy. Drizzle oil into yogurt, stirring constantly. Stir in vinegar, onion, parsley, and dill. Refrigerate.

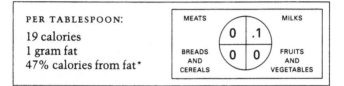

PER TABLESPOON:
19 calories
1 gram fat
47% calories from fat*

MEATS 0 | .1 MILKS
BREADS AND CEREALS 0 | 0 FRUITS AND VEGETABLES

YOGURT-DILL SAUCE

You can save up to 30 grams of fat if you use our dill sauce rather than 100 percent-fat commercial dill sauce.

Makes 2 cups

1 cup nonfat yogurt
1/2 teaspoon dried dill
1/2 teaspoon Dijon mustard

1/2 cup chopped green pepper
1/2 cup chopped green onion,
    including tops

Mix together all ingredients; chill well. Serve with fish.

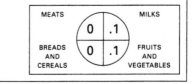

PER TABLESPOON:
10 calories
<1 gram fat
4% calories from fat

MEATS 0 | .1 MILKS
BREADS AND CEREALS 0 | .1 FRUITS AND VEGETABLES

* See p. 48, no. 2

CUCUMBER SAUCE

Another great use of the bounty of summer cucumbers. This sauce is excellent with broiled fish.

Makes 1 cup

½ cup peeled, seeded cucumber
½ cup nonfat sour cream
1 tablespoon chopped chives

1 tablespoon chopped green
   onion
1 tablespoon lemon juice
¼ teaspoon salt

Shred cucumber and blot very dry with paper towel. Add rest of ingredients and mix well. Chill.

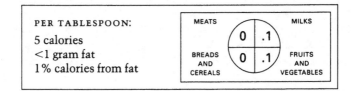

PER TABLESPOON:

5 calories
<1 gram fat
1% calories from fat

MEATS 0 | .1 MILKS
BREADS AND CEREALS 0 | .1 FRUITS AND VEGETABLES

21

Poultry

CHICKEN CURRY

Spicy and hot with cool undertones!

Serves 8

*8 boneless, skinless
    chicken-breast halves
1 cup nonfat plain yogurt
1 teaspoon curry powder
1/2 teaspoon ground cumin
dash salt
1/2 teaspoon garlic powder*

*1/4 teaspoon cayenne pepper
1 teaspoon oil
1 onion, chopped
2 cups chopped fresh tomatoes
1 teaspoon cornstarch
1 teaspoon water*

Mix together yogurt, curry powder, cumin, salt, garlic powder, and cayenne pepper. Coat chicken with this mixture and refrigerate for 4 hours.

Heat oil in nonstick skillet, add onion, and brown lightly. Stir in tomatoes and add chicken plus marinade. Mix well, cover, and simmer about 30 minutes.

If desired, thicken juices with 1 teaspoon cornstarch mixed with 1 teaspoon water.

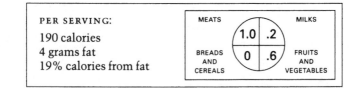

PER SERVING:
190 calories
4 grams fat
19% calories from fat

MEATS 1.0 | .2 MILKS
BREADS AND CEREALS 0 | .6 FRUITS AND VEGETABLES

CHICKEN WITH ORANGE SAUCE

When you remove the skin from chicken, you cut more than half the calories — and the cooking flavors are absorbed into the meat instead of the skin.

Serves 4

4 boneless, skinless
   chicken-breast halves
2 tablespoons vegetable oil
1 medium green pepper,
   chopped
1 cup fresh mushrooms,
   chopped

2 11-ounce cans mandarin
   oranges
²/₃ cup orange juice
¼ teaspoon powdered ginger
1 ½ tablespoons cornstarch
2 cups cooked brown rice

Cut chicken into bite-size pieces. Add oil to nonstick skillet; brown chicken for 1 minute, and remove from skillet. Add green pepper and mushrooms and cook just until tender. Drain oranges, saving syrup; add oranges to skillet. Place chicken back in skillet and cook until no pink shows when cut in thickest part (about 10 minutes). Blend ginger and cornstarch into mandarin-orange syrup and orange juice. Add to chicken and vegetable mixture. Heat, stirring until sauce thickens. Serve over rice.

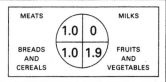

PER SERVING:
400 calories
11 grams fat
25% calories from fat

MEATS | MILKS
1.0 | 0
BREADS AND CEREALS | 1.0 | 1.9 | FRUITS AND VEGETABLES

ORANGE-AND-SPINACH-STUFFED CHICKEN BREASTS

Spinach and oranges? Surely there's been a mistake!! Not so — it's a delicious combination that complements the chicken!

Serves 6

*6 boneless, skinless chicken-
  breast halves*

STUFFING

*¾ cup cooked orzo
  (rice-shaped pasta)
1 10-ounce box frozen cut
  spinach
1 11-ounce can mandarin*

*oranges, drained, liquid
  reserved
¼ cup chopped onion
1 garlic clove, crushed
dash salt
¼ teaspoon pepper*

TARRAGON-ORANGE SAUCE

*⅔ cup orange juice
⅔ cup reserved mandarin-
  orange liquid*

*1 tablespoon cornstarch
1 teaspoon dried tarragon
¼ teaspoon salt*

Place one chicken-breast half between two pieces of plastic wrap or waxed paper. Working from center, gently pound chicken with rolling pin or flat side of meat mallet until about ¼-inch thick. Repeat with remaining chicken breast halves.

In medium-sized bowl, combine all stuffing ingredients; mix well. Place ⅓–½ cup stuffing mixture down center third of each chicken breast. Bring ends of breast over stuffing; fold in sides. Secure with toothpicks. Place stuffed chicken breasts, seam side down, in ungreased 12 × 8-inch (2-quart) baking dish.

Heat oven to 350 degrees. In small saucepan, combine all sauce ingredients; blend well. Bring to boil over medium-high heat. Cook 3–5 minutes or until sauce is thickened, stirring constantly. Pour over chicken. Bake at 350 degrees for 35–40 minutes or until chicken is fork-tender and juices run clear. Garnish with additional mandarin oranges and fresh tarragon, if desired.

Microwave Directions. Prepare chicken and stuffing as directed. Place stuffed chicken breasts in 12 × 8-inch (2-quart) microwave-safe baking dish. Set aside. In small microwave-safe bowl, combine all sauce ingredients; blend well. Microwave on high for 6–7 minutes or until sauce thickens, stirring twice during cooking. Pour sauce over chicken; cover with waxed paper. Microwave on high for 15–20 minutes or until chicken is fork-tender and juices run clear, rearranging chicken halfway through cooking.

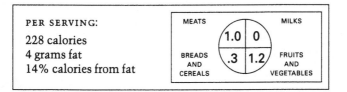

PER SERVING:

228 calories
4 grams fat
14% calories from fat

MEATS 1.0 | MILKS 0
BREADS AND CEREALS .3 | 1.2 FRUITS AND VEGETABLES

If you make poor choices about the way you eat and exercise, you can't blame your children for doing what you do. If you tell them it's important to eat a balanced diet, and they see you eating lots of greasy snacks or having drinks every night before dinner, your integrity is going to go down the drain.

BAKED CHICKEN WITH VEGETABLES

A bed of creamy vegetables is the perfect complement for this sea-soned chicken.

Serves 4

CHICKEN

2 tablespoons reduced-calorie
  margarine, melted
1/4 teaspoon dried tarragon
  leaves, optional

4 boneless, skinless
  chicken-breast halves

VEGETABLES

3/4 cup water
1 16-ounce package mixed
  frozen broccoli, cauliflower,
  and carrots
2 tablespoons reduced-calorie
  margarine, melted
2 tablespoons flour

1/4 teaspoon salt
1/8 teaspoon pepper
3/4 cup nonfat milk
2 tablespoons white wine
1 tablespoon Dijon mustard
sliced almonds

Heat oven to 375 degrees. In small bowl, combine margarine and tarragon. Place chicken breasts in ungreased 8- or 9-inch-square pan; brush with margarine mixture. Cover with foil. Bake at 375 degrees for 50 minutes or until chicken is fork-tender and juices run clear.

Meanwhile, in medium-sized saucepan bring 3/4 cup water to a boil; add frozen vegetables. Bring to a second boil, stir, cover, and reduce heat. Simmer 5–7 minutes or until vegetables are crisp-tender, stirring once during cooking. Remove vegetables with slotted spoon, and set aside. Pour vegetable liquid into a separate container. In same saucepan, combine margarine, flour, salt, and pepper; blend well. Cook over low heat until mixture is smooth and bubbly. Stir in milk. Cook over medium heat, stirring constantly, until mixture boils and thickens. If too thick, dilute with reserved vegetable liq-uid. Stir in wine, mustard, and warm vegetables; heat thoroughly.

Arrange cooked chicken breasts and vegetables on serving platter; sprinkle with almonds.

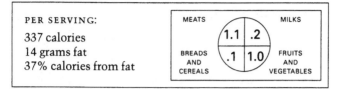

PER SERVING:		
337 calories		
14 grams fat		
37% calories from fat		

	MEATS	MILKS
	1.1	.2
BREADS AND CEREALS	.1	1.0
		FRUITS AND VEGETABLES

GRILLED GARLIC-PEPPER CHICKEN

You'll love the combination of flavors in this recipe.

Serves 5

1 cup white wine or chicken broth
2 tablespoons olive oil
1 teaspoon dried cilantro
1 teaspoon coarsely ground black pepper

½ teaspoon salt
6 garlic cloves, crushed
1 hot pepper, seeded and chopped
1 2½–3-pound chicken, skinned and cut up

In small bowl, combine all ingredients except chicken; blend well. Place chicken pieces in large nonmetal bowl or plastic bag; pour marinade over chicken. Cover bowl or seal bag; refrigerate. Marinate at least 30 minutes or up to several hours, turning chicken several times.

Heat grill and lightly oil grill rack. Drain chicken, reserving marinade. Place chicken pieces on gas grill, using indirect medium-high heat, or on charcoal grill 4–6 inches above medium-high coals. Cook for 30–40 minutes or until chicken is fork-tender and juices run clear, brushing with marinade and turning twice during cooking.

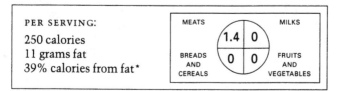

PER SERVING:		
250 calories		
11 grams fat		
39% calories from fat*		

	MEATS	MILKS
	1.4	0
BREADS AND CEREALS	0	0
		FRUITS AND VEGETABLES

* See p. 48, no. 2.

ITALIAN FRIED CHICKEN

A serving of regular fried chicken has 6 grams of fat and 40–50 percent fat calories.

Serves 6

*6 boneless, skinless
    chicken-breast halves
2 egg whites
2 tablespoons water
⅓ cup cornmeal*

*salt and pepper
1 teaspoon dried oregano or 1
    tablespoon fresh oregano
¾ cup nonfat mozzarella
    cheese, shredded*

Heat oven to 350 degrees. On hard surface, pound chicken with meat mallet or rolling pin to ¼-inch thickness. Heat nonstick skillet coated with nonstick cooking spray on medium heat. Mix egg whites and water; dip breasts in egg mixture, allowing excess to drip off. Dip in cornmeal and shake off excess. Place in skillet a few pieces at a time. Brown on both sides, about 3 minutes altogether. Remove from heat. Spray shallow baking dish with a light coat of nonstick cooking spray. Arrange chicken in dish. Sprinkle with salt, pepper, and oregano. Top with shredded cheese. Cover with foil and bake at 350 degrees for 15 minutes. Remove foil and continue baking until nicely browned, 15–20 minutes.

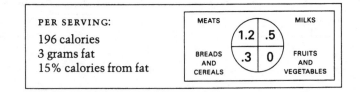

PER SERVING:
196 calories
3 grams fat
15% calories from fat

MEATS 1.2 | MILKS .5
BREADS AND CEREALS .3 | FRUITS AND VEGETABLES 0

CHICKEN SUCCOTASH

Succotash was not one of my favorite dishes — *until* I tried this one!

Serves 4

⅓ cup finely ground nonfat
   pepper crackers
1 pound boneless, skinless
   chicken breast, sliced into
   2-inch strips
1 tablespoon canola or olive oil
½ cup nonfat milk
4 ounces nonfat cream cheese

1 10-ounce box frozen lima
   beans, thawed and drained
1 10-ounce package frozen
   corn, thawed and drained
½ cup sliced green onion
1 teaspoon Tabasco or other
   hot pepper sauce

Put cracker crumbs and chicken pieces in plastic bag and shake until pieces are well coated. In large nonstick skillet, heat oil over medium heat; add chicken and cook about 10 minutes or until no longer pink. While chicken is cooking, blend milk and cream cheese; place in nonstick saucepan along with lima beans, corn, and green onion. Heat until almost boiling, then reduce heat and simmer until green onions are tender. Add hot pepper sauce and stir; spoon over chicken.

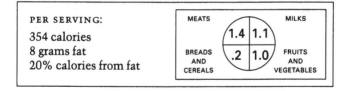

PER SERVING:
354 calories
8 grams fat
20% calories from fat

MEATS   1.4 | 1.1   MILKS
BREADS AND CEREALS   .2 | 1.0   FRUITS AND VEGETABLES

CHICKEN CHASSEUR

You can substitute 1 cup of white wine for 1 cup of the chicken broth.

Serves 8

2½ pounds boneless, skinless chicken breast
½ cup flour
3 tablespoons corn oil
1 pound whole mushrooms
1 medium onion, chopped

1 ½ cups defatted chicken broth
1 cup tomato sauce
1 tablespoon Kitchen Bouquet seasoning
juice of one lemon
¼ cup chopped fresh parsley

Heat oven to 325 degrees. Dredge chicken in flour. Brown in oil in nonstick pan, then transfer to an 8½ x 14-inch casserole. Add mushrooms and onions to skillet and sauté; slowly add chicken broth, tomato sauce, Kitchen Bouquet, and lemon juice. Pour sauce over chicken. Bake at 325 degrees for 45 minutes. Serve over cooked rice. Garnish with parsley.

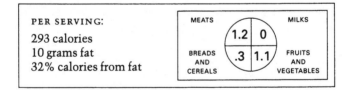

PER SERVING:
293 calories
10 grams fat
32% calories from fat

| MEATS | 1.2 | 0 | MILKS |
| BREADS AND CEREALS | .3 | 1.1 | FRUITS AND VEGETABLES |

*P*eople with healthy attitudes know that they're going to eat — it's just a question of what and when. What a shame that many people don't think about exercise the same way. Healthy people know they're going to exercise, just as they know they're going to eat.

ORIENTAL CHICKEN STIR-FRY

You can use frozen cut vegetables in this dish to shorten preparation time. Thaw them first or cook a few minutes longer.

Serves 4

2 boneless, skinless
  chicken-breast halves
1 tablespoon oil
3 garlic cloves, crushed
2 cups mixed vegetables, your
  choice

⅓ cup chopped green onion
¼ cup red plum jelly
2 tablespoons soy sauce
2 tablespoons white wine or
  chicken broth
2 teaspoons cornstarch

Cut chicken into ½-inch pieces. Heat large skillet or wok over medium-high heat until hot. Add oil; heat until it ripples. Add chicken and garlic; cook 5–6 minutes or until chicken is no longer pink, stirring constantly. Stir in mixed vegetables and green onion. Cook 5–8 minutes or until vegetables are crisp-tender, stirring frequently. Stir in plum jelly and soy sauce. In a small bowl, combine white wine and cornstarch; blend well. Stir cornstarch mixture into hot chicken mixture. Cook and stir 1–3 minutes or until slightly thickened and glaze covers all ingredients. Serve with hot cooked rice if desired.

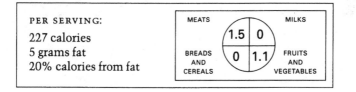

PER SERVING:
227 calories
5 grams fat
20% calories from fat

MEATS 1.5 | 0 MILKS
BREADS AND CEREALS 0 | 1.1 FRUITS AND VEGETABLES

HUNGARIAN-STYLE CHICKEN PAPRIKA

This is my mom's original—defatted from 67 percent to 19 percent fat calories.

Serves 10

1 tablespoon canola oil
2 large onions, chopped
3 tablespoons paprika,
  preferably Hungarian
3 ½ pounds boneless, skinless
  chicken breast, cut into
  pieces

1 28-ounce can stewed
  tomatoes, undrained
dash salt
2 tablespoons flour
1 cup nonfat sour cream
4 cups cooked rice

Heat oven to 250 degrees. Put oil in large nonstick skillet, add onions, and sauté until golden brown; add paprika and mix well into the onions. Add chicken pieces, stewed tomatoes, and salt; cover and simmer over low heat until chicken is tender. Remove chicken to an 8½ × 14-inch casserole. Add flour to any juices in the pan, then, 1 tablespoon at a time, add thickened juices to sour cream. Return mixture to skillet and cook over very low heat, stirring, until hot. Pour over chicken. Cover casserole, put in oven, and cook at 250 degrees for 30 minutes. Serve over rice.

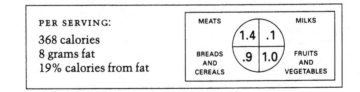

PER SERVING:
368 calories
8 grams fat
19% calories from fat

MEATS 1.4 | .1 MILKS
BREADS AND CEREALS .9 | 1.0 FRUITS AND VEGETABLES

CHICKEN STEW

This is another easy-to-prepare dish that makes good use of an overflowing vegetable garden.

Serves 4

1 pound boneless, skinless
  chicken breast, cut into
  chunks
2 cups cooked rice
2 medium tomatoes, cut into
  chunks
1 cup halved fresh mushrooms

1 medium zucchini, sliced in
  1-inch rounds
2 cloves garlic, minced
1 tablespoon chopped fresh
  basil
fresh ground pepper to taste

Combine chicken with other ingredients in a 3½-quart slow cooker; stir well. Cook on medium-high setting at least 3 hours. Reduce heat for last 30 minutes.

PER SERVING:

286 calories
5 grams fat
16% calories from fat

MEATS		MILKS
1.0	0	
BREADS AND CEREALS		FRUITS AND VEGETABLES
1.0	1.2	

CROCK-POT CHICKEN

The chicken practically falls off the bone in this dish.

Serves 8

3–4-pound chicken, cut up, skin removed
salt and pepper
½ cup chopped green onion
½ cup soy sauce
¼ cup dry white wine
½ cup water
¼ cup honey
2 cups uncooked brown rice

Sprinkle chicken with salt and pepper. Put all ingredients except rice in a slow cooker; cook 3–4 hours on high. With one hour to go, cook rice according to package directions. Serve chicken pieces on top of rice and cover with sauce left in slow cooker.

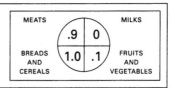

PER SERVING:
280 calories
5 grams fat
18% calories from fat

MEATS .9   MILKS 0
BREADS AND CEREALS 1.0   FRUITS AND VEGETABLES .1

CHINESE CHICKEN PIZZA

This recipe came from Covert's secretary, Marni, and it is one of our favorites. The ingredients may seem unusual, but when your family sinks their teeth into this pizza you'll see smiles all around.

Serves 8

8 ounces boneless, skinless chicken breast, cut into cubes
2 tablespoons chunky peanut butter
4 cloves garlic, minced
1 tablespoon minced fresh ginger
¼ cup brown sugar
¾ cup white wine vinegar or rice wine vinegar
¼ cup soy sauce
⅛ teaspoon crushed red pepper
3 tablespoons water
½ cup shredded part-skim mozzarella cheese
1 large pizza crust

Heat oven to 450 degrees. Cook chicken in nonstick pan sprayed with nonfat cooking spray just until it is no longer pink. Remove from pan. Whisk next 8 ingredients together and add to pan. Cook over medium-high heat, stirring constantly. When sauce is bubbly and starts to thicken, return chicken to pan. Cook until semi-syrupy. Put grated cheese on pizza crust. Spread chicken mixture on top. Bake at 450 degrees about 10 minutes. Let stand 5 minutes.

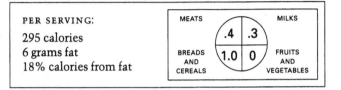

PER SERVING:
295 calories
6 grams fat
18% calories from fat

CHICKEN CARIB

This is a lot like fried chicken, but tastier.

Serves 4

1 pound boneless, skinless chicken breast
½ cup evaporated skim milk

1 envelope garlic-style salad dressing seasoning
1 cup crushed nonfat corn chips

Heat oven to 375 degrees. Dip chicken in evaporated skim milk, sprinkle with garlic seasoning, and roll in crushed chips. Place on foil-lined baking sheet and bake at 375 degrees for 20 minutes.

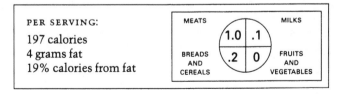

PER SERVING:
197 calories
4 grams fat
19% calories from fat

CHICKEN AND SALSA VERDE CASSEROLE

Serves 8

2 medium onions, diced
2 tablespoons chicken broth
2 cups diced cooked chicken
½ cup picante salsa
8 ounces nonfat cream cheese

12 6-inch corn tortillas
1 cup shredded nonfat sharp
  cheddar cheese
1 cup shredded part-skim
  mozzarella cheese

Cook onion in broth over medium heat until translucent and beginning to brown, about 20 minutes. Remove pan from heat and add chicken, salsa, and cream cheese; mix lightly. Heat oven to 350 degrees. Soften tortillas by wrapping in damp cloth and then in foil; bake at 350 degrees for about 10 minutes or until soft. Spray a 9 × 13-inch baking dish with nonstick cooking spray. Alternate layers of tortillas, chicken mixture, and cheese — finishing with tortillas and topping with cheese. Bake at 350 degrees for 30 minutes.

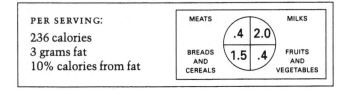

PER SERVING:
236 calories
3 grams fat
10% calories from fat

MEATS .4 2.0 MILKS
BREADS AND CEREALS 1.5 .4 FRUITS AND VEGETABLES

MEXICAN CHICKEN

Serves 6

1 medium onion, chopped
1 clove garlic, minced
1 cup V-8 juice
1 teaspoon basil
1 teaspoon oregano
1 teaspoon chili powder
3 cups boneless, skinless

cooked chicken breast, in
  chunks
1 small can chopped green
  chilies
½ cup grated low-fat cheddar
  cheese
½ cup fat-free corn chips,
  crushed

Combine onion, garlic, V-8 juice, and seasonings in saucepan; simmer for 1 hour. Heat oven to 350 degrees. In a 8½ × 14-inch baking

dish, layer the chicken, chilies and cheese; top with sauce. Sprinkle
with crushed tortillas. Bake at 350 degrees for 30 minutes.

PER SERVING:		
185 calories	MEATS	MILKS
5 grams fat	.8 .3	
22% calories from fat	BREADS AND CEREALS .2 .8	FRUITS AND VEGETABLES

CHICKEN ENCHILADAS

Serve this favorite with Spanish-style rice, and finish the meal with
Fruit and Yogurt Crunch Pops (page 211).

Serves 4

4 large corn tortillas
1 pound boneless, skinless
  chicken breast, cooked and
  chopped
8 ounces nonfat cream cheese

1 4-ounce can chopped green
  chilies
1 cup enchilada sauce
¼ cup nonfat mayonnaise
3 tablespoons water

Heat oven to 425 degrees. Stack tortillas and wrap in foil; place in
oven for 5 minutes. While tortillas heat, mix chicken, half the
cream cheese, and chilies in a medium-sized bowl. In a separate
bowl, combine enchilada sauce, mayonnaise, and water and stir
until smooth. Spread half of sauce mixture over bottom of nonstick
baking dish. Remove warm tortillas from oven. Spoon a heaping ⅓
cup chicken mixture down the center of each tortilla; roll tortilla
around the filling; place seam side down in baking dish. Pour remaining sauce mixture over top. Cover dish with foil. Bake 15
minutes or until very hot. Put dollops of remaining cream cheese on
top and bake uncovered 10 minutes or until cheese melts and sauce
bubbles around edges.

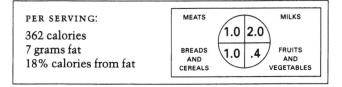

PER SERVING:		
362 calories	MEATS	MILKS
7 grams fat	1.0 2.0	
18% calories from fat	BREADS AND CEREALS 1.0 .4	FRUITS AND VEGETABLES

CHICKEN CACCIATORE

You can use mushrooms, zucchini, or eggplant instead of peppers and onion.

Serves 8

1 30-ounce jar prepared
   spaghetti sauce
½ cup burgundy or other dry
   red wine
1 medium onion, cut into
   1-inch pieces
1 medium green pepper, cut
   into 1-inch pieces

1½ pounds boneless, skinless
   chicken breast
1 teaspoon Italian herb
   seasoning
¼ teaspoon ground cumin
salt and pepper to taste
3½ cups cooked spinach
   fettuccine

Combine first 4 ingredients in Dutch oven or slow cooker; stir well. Add chicken breasts, stirring to coat. Place on medium-high heat and bring to a boil. Cover, reduce heat, and simmer 2 hours or until chicken is done. Remove chicken pieces; let cool. Add Italian seasoning, cumin, salt, and pepper to sauce mixture; stir well. Cover and cook over medium heat another 15 minutes, stirring occasionally. Cut chicken into bite-size pieces. Add to sauce mixture and heat thoroughly. Serve over fettuccine.

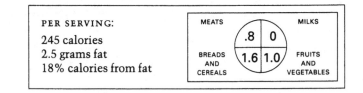

PER SERVING:
245 calories
2.5 grams fat
18% calories from fat

MEATS .8   MILKS 0
BREADS AND CEREALS 1.6   FRUITS AND VEGETABLES 1.0

TURKEY TETRAZZINI

Despite the long list of ingredients, this recipe is easy and fast, and it's a great way to use leftover turkey. To save time, start boiling the water for the spaghetti when you begin sautéing the mushrooms. Try it with macaroni or penne instead of spaghetti.

Serves 4

1½ cups sliced mushrooms
2 tablespoons flour
dash salt and pepper
2 cups nonfat milk
1 teaspoon Worcestershire
  sauce
½ cup shredded low-fat
  cheddar cheese

1 green pepper, diced
½ cup sliced scallions
2 pimientos, finely chopped
2 cups cooked turkey, cut into
  small cubes
½ pound spaghetti, cooked
  and drained
¼ cup grated Parmesan cheese

Heat oven to 350 degrees. In large nonstick skillet or microwave oven, cook mushrooms until tender. Stir in flour, salt, and pepper, then gradually add milk, stirring constantly to prevent lumps. Add Worcestershire sauce and simmer until somewhat thickened. Add cheese, green pepper, scallions, and pimientos and mix well; stir in turkey and spaghetti, combining well. Pour mixture into 2-quart shallow casserole or baking dish sprayed with nonstick cooking spray; sprinkle with Parmesan cheese. Bake casserole uncovered at 350 degrees for 20 minutes or until heated through.

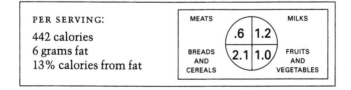

PER SERVING:
442 calories
6 grams fat
13% calories from fat

MEATS .6 | 1.2 MILKS
BREADS AND CEREALS 2.1 | 1.0 FRUITS AND VEGETABLES

TURKEY-NOODLE SCALLOP

For a change, try red or yellow pepper instead of green pepper.

Serves 4

⅓ cup minced onion
2 tablespoons minced green
   pepper
½ cup nonfat cream cheese
½ cup nonfat milk

½ cup shredded nonfat
   cheddar cheese
2 cups cooked noodles of your
   choice
2 cups diced cooked turkey

Heat oven to 400 degrees. Sauté onion and green pepper in nonstick pan sprayed with nonstick cooking spray. Meanwhile, mix cream cheese, milk, and cheddar cheese until well blended. Stir in onion-pepper mixture, noodles, and turkey. Put in baking dish and bake at 400 degrees for 20 minutes.

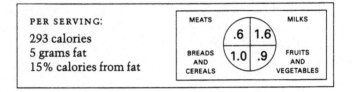

PER SERVING:

293 calories
5 grams fat
15% calories from fat

MEATS   MILKS
.6 1.6
BREADS   FRUITS
AND   1.0 .9   AND
CEREALS   VEGETABLES

HEARTY TURKEY CASSEROLE

This is a defatted variation of a popular hamburger casserole that calls for beef, sour cream, cream cheese, cheddar cheese, and cottage cheese. Fat cells love it! You'll find this version equally creamy but not nearly so rich.

Serves 4

1 pound lean ground turkey	*¾ cup low-fat cottage cheese*
1 onion, chopped	*¼ cup nonfat plain yogurt*
1 clove garlic, minced	*6 ounces noodles, cooked and*
½ teaspoon dried basil	*drained*
½ teaspoon dried oregano	*¾ cup shredded nonfat*
dash salt	*mozzarella cheese*
1 cup tomato sauce	

Heat oven to 350 degrees. Starting with a cold nonstick skillet, brown turkey slowly, breaking into small chunks. Drain off any fat. Add onion and garlic and cook for 2 minutes. Stir in spices and tomato sauce and heat briefly until sauce is thick and bubbling.

Meanwhile, blend together cottage cheese and yogurt until smooth. In a 9 × 13-inch baking dish, spread half the noodles in a thin layer. Top with half of the meat sauce and all of the cottage cheese mixture, then repeat the layers of noodles and meat. Top with mozzarella cheese.

Bake at 350 degrees for 45 minutes or until cheese is browned and casserole bubbles.

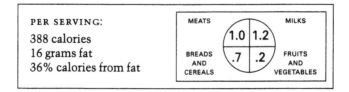

PER SERVING:
388 calories
16 grams fat
36% calories from fat

MEATS 1.0 | 1.2 MILKS
BREADS AND CEREALS .7 | .2 FRUITS AND VEGETABLES

TURKEY MEAT LOAF

I like this even better the day after, when I make cold meat loaf sandwiches.

Serves 4

1 pound ground turkey
½ cup crumbled nonfat
  crackers
¼ cup finely chopped onion
1 egg, beaten
1 tablespoon chicken broth or
  water

1 tablespoon Worcestershire
  sauce
½ teaspoon salt
½ teaspoon poultry seasoning
¼ cup tomato sauce
2 tablespoons water

Heat oven to 325 degrees. In a medium-sized bowl, combine all ingredients except tomato sauce and water. Pat into a 4 × 8-inch loaf pan and bake at 325 degrees for 1 hour. Mix together tomato sauce and water and baste meat loaf frequently with it.

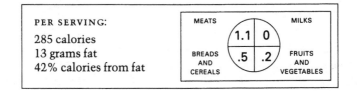

PER SERVING:

285 calories
13 grams fat
42% calories from fat

MEATS 1.1 MILKS 0
BREADS AND CEREALS .5 FRUITS AND VEGETABLES .2

TURKEY-ZUCCHINI LASAGNA

If you put this together and refrigerate ahead of time, you can just pop it into the oven when you come home.

Serves 6

5 ounces ground turkey
⅓ cup chopped onion
1 15-ounce can tomato sauce
½ teaspoon oregano
¼ teaspoon basil
⅛ teaspoon pepper

6 medium zucchini
2 tablespoons flour
1 cup low-fat cottage cheese
(1%)
¼ cup nonfat shredded
mozzarella cheese

In a 10-inch skillet over medium heat, cook ground turkey and onion until tender, about 10 minutes, stirring occasionally. Drain any fat. Add tomato sauce, oregano, basil, and pepper; heat to boiling. Reduce heat to low and simmer 5 minutes, stirring occasionally.

Heat oven to 375 degrees. Slice zucchini lengthwise into ¼-inch-thick slices. In bottom of a 12 × 8-inch baking dish, arrange half the zucchini in a layer and sprinkle with 1 tablespoon flour. Top with cottage cheese and half of meat mixture. Repeat with remaining zucchini and flour; sprinkle with mozzarella cheese and then remaining meat mixture. Bake at 375 degrees for 40 minutes or until hot and bubbly and zucchini is fork-tender. Let stand 10 minutes for easier cutting.

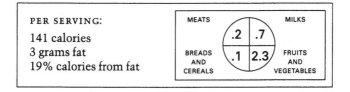

PER SERVING:
141 calories
3 grams fat
19% calories from fat

MEATS .2 | .7 MILKS
BREADS AND CEREALS .1 | 2.3 FRUITS AND VEGETABLES

FRITTATA FOR FOUR

This is great for lunch or a light dinner. Use whatever vegetables you have on hand.

Serves 4

1 teaspoon oil
1½ cups assorted sliced raw
 vegetables
6 ounces diced turkey-ham
½ cup nonfat milk
3 eggs

2 egg whites
¼ cup grated part-skim
 mozzarella
¼ cup grated low-fat sharp
 cheddar cheese

Heat oven to 350 degrees. Heat oil in nonstick skillet; add vegetables and brown until crisp-tender. Add turkey-ham and warm. Beat together milk, eggs, and egg whites; stir in cheeses and pour over vegetable–turkey-ham mixture. Pour into 1-quart casserole dish coated with nonstick cooking spray and bake at 350 degrees for 20 minutes.

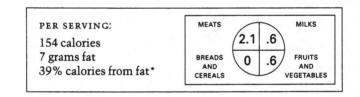

PER SERVING:
154 calories
7 grams fat
39% calories from fat*

MEATS   MILKS
2.1   .6
BREADS AND CEREALS   0   .6   FRUITS AND VEGETABLES

* See p. 47, no. 1.

22

Vegetables and Side Dishes

ASPARAGUS IN ORANGE SAUCE

This recipe sounds weird, but it works. Try serving it with chicken and rice. You can use fresh asparagus instead of canned: snap off tough ends and cook in a steamer or microwave.

Serves 3

1 15-ounce can asparagus,   2 teaspoons cornstarch
   drained, reserving liquid   ½ cup orange juice
1 tablespoon honey

Heat asparagus slowly in saucepan. Combine honey, cornstarch, and orange juice in a small pan. Heat slowly, stirring constantly. If you need more liquid, use the reserve from the asparagus. Spoon sauce over asparagus to serve.

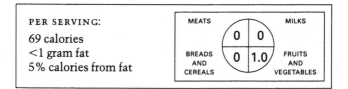

PER SERVING:
69 calories
<1 gram fat
5% calories from fat

MEATS 0 | MILKS 0
BREADS AND CEREALS 0 | 1.0 FRUITS AND VEGETABLES

BARBECUE GREEN BEANS

This is my favorite kind of recipe. Mix, serve, and take the accolades for your creativity.

Serves 6

4 cups cooked green beans,   1 cup barbecue sauce with
   drained   onions

Combine and heat!

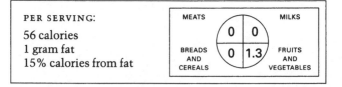

PER SERVING:
56 calories
1 gram fat
15% calories from fat

MEATS 0 | MILKS 0
BREADS AND CEREALS 0 | 1.3 FRUITS AND VEGETABLES

DEVILED GREEN BEANS

Hot and spicy finger food well suited to fresh green beans.

Serves 6

4 cups cooked extra-large green
   beans
1 teaspoon Dijon mustard
1 teaspoon Worcestershire
   sauce

dash seasoned salt
⅛ teaspoon pepper
dash cayenne pepper

Combine all ingredients in saucepan, stir well, and heat. Chill before serving.

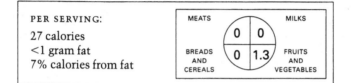

PER SERVING:
27 calories
<1 gram fat
7% calories from fat

MEATS 0   MILKS 0
BREADS AND CEREALS 0   FRUITS AND VEGETABLES 1.3

GREEN BEANS WITH SOUR CREAM

This tastes best when made with fresh green beans, but if you want to save time, use canned or frozen beans instead.

Serves 6

1 cup sliced mushrooms
½ teaspoon oil
4 cups cooked green beans

dash seasoned salt
⅛ teaspoon pepper
1 cup nonfat sour cream

Sauté mushrooms in oil in nonstick pan. Add beans, salt, and pepper. Slowly add nonfat sour cream and heat thoroughly.

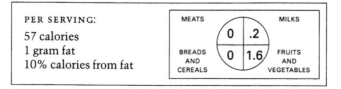

PER SERVING:
57 calories
1 gram fat
10% calories from fat

MEATS 0   MILKS .2
BREADS AND CEREALS 0   FRUITS AND VEGETABLES 1.6

GREEN BEANS WITH CHEESE

Only 4 percent fat calories instead of the 73 percent in the original version.

Serves 6

4 cups cooked green beans, drained
1/3 cup nonfat cream cheese
1/4 cup nonfat milk

3/4 cup grated nonfat cheddar cheese
dash seasoned salt
1/8 teaspoon cayenne pepper

Heat oven to 350 degrees. In small saucepan, warm cream cheese over low heat and mix with milk until creamy; stir in 1/2 cup grated cheese. Arrange beans in nonstick baking dish or casserole; sprinkle with salt and cayenne; stir in cheese mixture. Bake in oven for 15 minutes. Remove and sprinkle with remaining grated cheese.

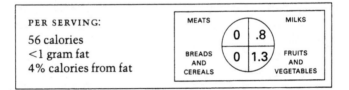

PER SERVING:
56 calories
<1 gram fat
4% calories from fat

MEATS 0 | .8 MILKS
BREADS AND CEREALS 0 | 1.3 FRUITS AND VEGETABLES

BEETS IN ORANGE SAUCE

Yes, I have a thing for orange juice — it heightens the flavor of most vegetables.

Serves 8

2 tablespoons cornstarch
3/4 cup orange juice
1 1/2 teaspoons grated orange rind

dash salt
1/4 teaspoon pepper
2 teaspoons sugar
4 cups sliced cooked beets

Mix cornstarch into orange juice, stirring well to avoid lumps. Add grated orange rind. Season with salt, pepper, and sugar. Heat slowly, add beets and heat thoroughly.

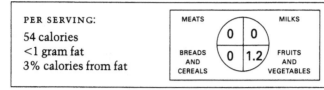

PER SERVING:
54 calories
<1 gram fat
3% calories from fat

MEATS 0 | MILKS 0
BREADS AND CEREALS 0 | FRUITS AND VEGETABLES 1.2

GLAZED CARROTS

To shorten the preparation time, I've used a variety of jams (4 teaspoons) instead of brown sugar and orange rind.

Serves 6

¾ pound whole baby carrots or
*   regular carrots cut small*
1 teaspoon water
2 teaspoons brown sugar

2 teaspoons grated orange rind
½ teaspoon dried dill
1 teaspoon powdered ginger

Steam carrots for 15 minutes or until barely tender. In a medium-sized skillet, mix water, brown sugar, orange rind, and dried dill. Add carrots and toss. Sprinkle with ginger and toss again. Cook 1–2 minutes or until carrots are lightly glazed. Serve.

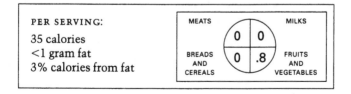

PER SERVING:
35 calories
<1 gram fat
3% calories from fat

MEATS 0 | MILKS 0
BREADS AND CEREALS 0 | FRUITS AND VEGETABLES .8

HOT PICKLED CARROTS

Dark, rich-tasting balsamic vinegar transforms ordinary recipes into extraordinary delights.

Serves 6

1⅓ pounds carrots, peeled and diced
¼ cup minced onion

3 tablespoons balsamic vinegar
1 bay leaf
salt and pepper

Mix carrots and onion in 1-quart casserole. Add vinegar and bay leaf; cover with lid and microwave on high for 5 minutes. Stir, cover with paper towel, and continue to cook until carrots are tender and almost all liquid has evaporated. Add salt and pepper to taste.

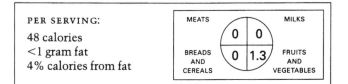

PER SERVING:
48 calories
<1 gram fat
4% calories from fat

MEATS			MILKS
	0	0	
BREADS AND CEREALS	0	1.3	FRUITS AND VEGETABLES

*W*hen I was a college professor, one of my students became so enamored of carrots that he practically lived on them. The palms of his hands and soles of his feet actually turned yellow! He was clearly going beyond the boundaries of reason, but he felt that if vitamin A and carotene are good for the body, then a lot must be very good.

SWEET CARROTS

Sweet and spicy — this is a great way to get beta carotene.

Serves 6

36 baby carrots (2 pounds)	*dash salt*
1 teaspoon butter	*⅓ teaspoon cinnamon*
½ cup sugar	*⅓ cup boiling water*

Heat oven to 350 degrees. Place carrots in casserole dish. Mix together butter, sugar, salt, and cinnamon; add water and blend well. Pour over carrots; cover and bake at 350 degrees for 1 hour.

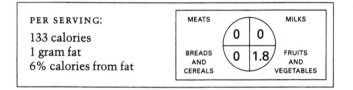

PER SERVING:
133 calories
1 gram fat
6% calories from fat

MEATS — 0
MILKS — 0
BREADS AND CEREALS — 0
FRUITS AND VEGETABLES — 1.8

I have to laugh at some of my health-nut friends who think that scraping a carrot removes all its vitamins. In its natural state, vitamin A is a yellow/orange carotene. It isn't removed by scraping the surface of a carrot. In fact, you can scrape all the way through and never run out of carotene.

BROILED CORN

Serves 6

8 tablespoons nonfat cream
  cheese, softened
1 tablespoon nonfat milk
4 cups cooked corn, fresh-cut
  or canned

dash salt
⅛ teaspoon pepper
½ cup grated nonfat cheddar
  cheese

Mix cream cheese and milk. Place corn in nonstick baking dish or casserole. Sprinkle with salt and pepper, then dot with cream cheese mixture; sprinkle with grated cheese. Place 7 inches below broiler flame for about 20 minutes or until cheese melts and top is brown.

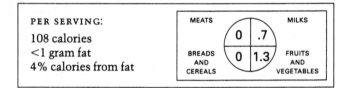

PER SERVING:
108 calories
<1 gram fat
4% calories from fat

	MEATS	MILKS
	0	.7
	BREADS AND CEREALS	FRUITS AND VEGETABLES
	0	1.3

DIJON MUSHROOMS AND ONIONS

For a milder flavor, replace the hot sauce with more Dijon mustard. For a very mild flavor, use regular mustard.

Serves 4

3 tablespoons water
2 teaspoons hot sauce
2 teaspoons Dijon mustard
½ teaspoon paprika
1 large onion, thinly sliced and
  separated into rings

1½ cups sliced fresh
  mushrooms
1 tablespoon low-sodium soy
  sauce

Combine water, hot sauce, Dijon mustard, and paprika in a large bowl; stir well. Add onion rings and coat gently. Coat a large nonstick skillet with nonstick cooking spray; place over medium heat until hot. Add onion mixture; cook 5 minutes, stirring constantly. Add mushrooms and cook 5 minutes or until mushrooms are tender, stirring constantly. Stir in soy sauce, cover, reduce heat, and simmer 1 minute. Serve piping hot.

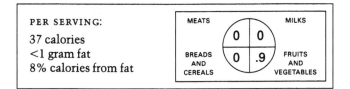

PER SERVING:
37 calories
<1 gram fat
8% calories from fat

MEATS 0 | 0 MILKS
BREADS AND CEREALS 0 | .9 FRUITS AND VEGETABLES

CONFETTI CORN

Colorful and as full of fireworks as the Fourth of July.

Serves 4

1 teaspoon oil
½ cup finely chopped onion
1 clove garlic, minced
½ cup finely chopped green
  pepper

½ cup finely chopped red
  pepper
2 cups whole-kernel corn
½ teaspoon ground cumin

Heat oil in nonstick skillet and add all other ingredients. Stir briefly, add salt and pepper to taste, cover, and cook over low heat about 3 minutes.

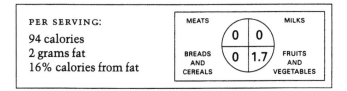

PER SERVING:
94 calories
2 grams fat
16% calories from fat

MEATS 0 | 0 MILKS
BREADS AND CEREALS 0 | 1.7 FRUITS AND VEGETABLES

MUSHROOMS WITH SOUR CREAM

Using nonfat sour cream cuts 8 grams of fat from each serving.

Serves 4

1 medium onion, diced fine	*1 teaspoon paprika*
1 tablespoon olive oil	*1 teaspoon lemon juice*
1 pound mushrooms, sliced	*1½ cups nonfat sour cream*
dash salt and freshly ground	
* black pepper*	

Sauté onion in olive oil in nonstick pan. Add mushrooms and sauté until tender but not limp or shriveled. Add rest of ingredients and heat *very* gently but thoroughly.

```
PER SERVING:              MEATS              MILKS

123 calories                   0  | .4
4 grams fat               BREADS            FRUITS
28% calories from fat     AND     0  | 1.3  AND
                          CEREALS           VEGETABLES
```

FRENCH PEAS

Try this sweet side dish in place of potatoes.

Serves 4

2 cups frozen peas	*¼ teaspoon sugar*
6 tiny white onions, peeled	*¼ cup water*
5–6 lettuce leaves, shredded	*1 teaspoon cornstarch*
3 sprigs parsley, tied with string	*1 teaspoon Molly McButter*
dash salt	

In saucepan, combine frozen peas, onions, lettuce leaves, parsley, salt and sugar. Mix together and add water. Cover and cook over medium heat until half the liquid is absorbed. Drain liquid into a small bowl and mix with cornstarch until smooth. Return to peas and stir well. Remove parsley, sprinkle peas with Molly McButter, and serve.

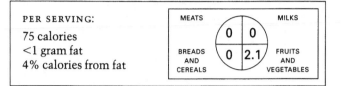

PER SERVING:
75 calories
<1 gram fat
4% calories from fat

MEATS 0 0 MILKS
BREADS AND CEREALS 0 2.1 FRUITS AND VEGETABLES

BAKED ACORN SQUASH

A single serving will give you all the vitamin A you need for the day.

Serves 2

*1 acorn squash, cut in half
  lengthwise and seeded*

*Molly McButter
nutmeg to taste*

Bake squash cut side down on aluminum foil or baking sheet at 350 degrees for 45 minutes or until tender. Season with Molly McButter and sprinkle with ground nutmeg.

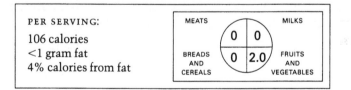

PER SERVING:
106 calories
<1 gram fat
4% calories from fat

MEATS 0 0 MILKS
BREADS AND CEREALS 0 2.0 FRUITS AND VEGETABLES

ZINGY STUFFED ZUCCHINI

This dish takes a little extra time to prepare, but it's well worth it. With a salad and some fresh hot bread, this "side dish" makes a good low-fat, high-fiber meal.

Serves 6

6 medium zucchini	*1 cup cooked brown rice*
1 clove garlic, split in half	*½ teaspoon dried oregano*
½ teaspoon margarine	*¼ teaspoon cayenne pepper*
1 medium onion, chopped	*salt and pepper*
1 cup chopped fresh tomatoes	*½ cup grated Parmesan cheese*

Wash zucchini, cut off stems, and cut in half lengthwise. In a small amount of boiling water, cook the zucchini, covered, for 5 minutes or until tender. Drain well, cool, and scoop out the seeds. Heat oven to 450 degrees. Sauté garlic in margarine until golden; lift out and discard garlic pieces. Add onion and sauté, stirring, until golden. Add tomatoes, rice, oregano, and cayenne; toss with fork to mix well. Sprinkle inside of each zucchini with salt and pepper. Place a portion of rice mixture inside each zucchini; sprinkle the top with Parmesan cheese. Arrange in a single layer in baking dish. Bake at 450 degrees, uncovered, for 15 minutes. Place under the broiler several minutes to brown the top. *Be careful not to burn!*

PER SERVING:	MEATS		MILKS
110 calories		0 .2	
3 grams fat	BREADS AND CEREALS	.3 1.9	FRUITS AND VEGETABLES
22% calories from fat			

FOUR-COLOR VEGGIES

For variety, use a nonfat salad dressing instead of the soy or Oriental sauce.

Serves 4

*1 10-ounce package frozen
    green peas
4 green onions, chopped
8 large mushrooms, sliced*

*16 cherry tomatoes, cut in half
1 tablespoon soy sauce or
    Yoshida Oriental gourmet
    sauce*

Cook peas according to package directions. Meanwhile, coat a non-stick frying pan with cooking spray and sauté the green onions and mushrooms until tender. Add tomatoes and stir. Add peas and toss with soy sauce.

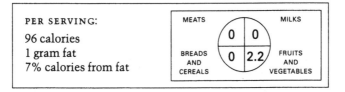

PER SERVING:

96 calories
1 gram fat
7% calories from fat

MEATS	MILKS
0	0
BREADS AND CEREALS	FRUITS AND VEGETABLES
0	2.2

I like the butter substitutes such as Butter Buds and Molly McButter. They add butter flavor to steamed vegetables without the butter calories. If you can fool me with something as obvious as butter on corn on the cob, it must be a good product!

GRILLED VEGETABLES WITH BASIL SAUCE

This vegetarian dish even has some Meat-group nutrients. Can you figure out where they come from?

Serves 6

2 egg whites	1 red pepper, quartered
5 teaspoons lemon juice	1 green or yellow pepper,
1 teaspoon Dijon mustard	quartered
¾ cup fresh basil leaves	1 zucchini, cut in ¼-inch
dash salt	rounds
¼ teaspoon white pepper	1 yellow squash, cut in ¼-inch
2 tablespoons olive oil	rounds
6 green onions, cut in 1-inch	8 mushrooms
pieces	wooden skewers soaked in
8 cherry tomatoes	water for 20 minutes

In a food processor or blender, blend egg whites, lemon juice, mustard, basil, salt, and pepper. Add the oil in a stream, blending the mixture until it thickens. This can be made a day in advance.

Thread the vegetables on wooden skewers and brush with basil sauce so they do not stick to grill. Grill over glowing coals, turning once.

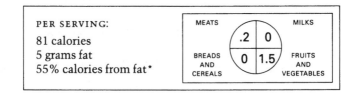

PER SERVING:
81 calories
5 grams fat
55% calories from fat*

MEATS .2   0 MILKS
BREADS AND CEREALS 0 | 1.5 FRUITS AND VEGETABLES

* See p. 48, no. 2.

TWICE-BAKED POTATOES

Sprinkle herbs, diced vegetables, or shredded cheese over the top.

Serves 4

*4 medium-sized baking
   potatoes
1 cup low-fat (1%) cottage
   cheese
½ cup nonfat milk or low-fat
   buttermilk
2 tablespoons minced onion*

*1 tablespoon dried parsley
   flakes
¼ teaspoon pepper
1 teaspoon Molly McButter or
   Butter Buds
salt to taste*

Scrub potatoes under cold water. Make shallow slits in each potato. Bake at 400 degrees for 45 minutes or until tender. Slice hot potatoes in half lengthwise. Spoon out potato, leaving skin intact for refilling. Beat remaining ingredients with a wire whisk until fluffy. Salt to taste. Stuff mixture back into skins. Bake 10 minutes more or until just golden.

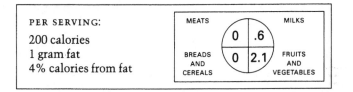

PER SERVING:

200 calories
1 gram fat
4% calories from fat

	MEATS		MILKS
	0	.6	
	BREADS AND CEREALS	FRUITS AND VEGETABLES	
	0	2.1	

What is it about baked potatoes that makes everyone say they're fattening? The chives, right?

SAVORY MICROWAVE RED POTATOES

Potatoes give you about 30 percent of the vitamin C you need for the day.

Serves 5

10 red potatoes, quartered	*2–4 tablespoons grated*
½ cup sliced leeks	*Parmesan cheese*
¼ cup chopped red pepper	

Spray 2-quart microwave-safe casserole with nonstick cooking spray. Add potatoes, leeks, and red pepper. Cover tightly. Microwave on high for 6–8 minutes or until potatoes are tender. Stir once halfway through cooking. Sprinkle with Parmesan cheese.

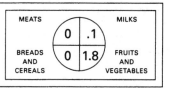

PER SERVING:
131 calories
1 gram fat
5% calories from fat

MEATS 0 | .1 MILKS
BREADS AND CEREALS 0 | 1.8 FRUITS AND VEGETABLES

ORANGE-PINEAPPLE SWEET POTATOES

Vitamin A is stored in the body. This recipe contains enough vitamin A to last you three days!

Serves 6

1½ cups hot cooked sweet potatoes, peeled	*reduced-calorie orange marmalade*
2 cups sliced hot cooked carrots	*1 teaspoon grated orange rind*
1 cup canned crushed pineapple (no sugar added)	*¼ teaspoon ground cinnamon*
2 tablespoons plus 2 teaspoons	*dash salt*

Heat oven to 375 degrees. Mash potatoes and carrots together, add remaining ingredients, and stir to combine. Put into a small casserole dish and bake at 375 degrees for 30 minutes.

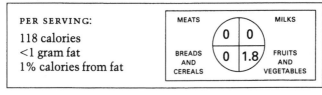

PER SERVING:	MEATS		MILKS
118 calories		0	0
<1 gram fat	BREADS AND CEREALS	0	1.8	FRUITS AND VEGETABLES
1% calories from fat			

PAPRIKA POTATOES

Add garlic or herbs to vary this recipe.

Serves 4

1 medium-sized onion, sliced
1 tablespoon olive oil
dash salt
1/8 teaspoon pepper

1/2 teaspoon paprika
4 medium-sized unpeeled red
   potatoes, sliced

Sauté onion in olive oil in nonstick pan until soft. During cooking, sprinkle with salt, pepper, and paprika. Add potatoes and enough water to cover them; cook until soft *but not mushy.*

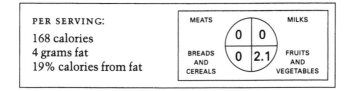

PER SERVING:	MEATS		MILKS
168 calories		0	0
4 grams fat	BREADS AND CEREALS	0	2.1	FRUITS AND VEGETABLES
19% calories from fat			

RISI E BISI (ITALIAN RICE AND PEAS)

This dish is delicious on its own and can also be made with additional vegetables and different seasonings.

Serves 1

½ cup hot firm-cooked brown
   rice
¼ cup boiling water
1 envelope instant chicken
   broth and seasoning mix

½ teaspoon dehydrated onion
   flakes
1 teaspoon minced parsley
pepper to taste
few drops sherry extract
½ cup uncooked peas

Combine all ingredients in small saucepan. Bring to a boil, reduce heat, cover, and simmer 15 minutes or until peas are soft. If peas and rice are too moist, remove cover and continue cooking.

PER SERVING:				
180 calories	MEATS 0	0	MILKS	
1 gram fat	BREADS AND CEREALS 1.0	1.1	FRUITS AND VEGETABLES	
5% calories from fat				

SPANISH RICE (MADE WITH RISI E BISI)

Serves 2

Risi e Bisi (p. 186 — double the recipe)

¾ cup V-8 juice
*½ teaspoon Worcestershire
    sauce*
½ medium green pepper, diced

1 ½ teaspoons diced pimiento
½ cup diced celery
dash Cayenne pepper

Combine all ingredients, including Risi e Bisi, in saucepan. Cook until vegetables are tender.

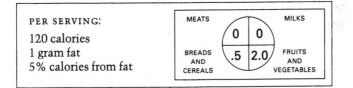

PER SERVING:
120 calories
1 gram fat
5% calories from fat

MEATS   MILKS
0   0
BREADS AND CEREALS   .5   2.0   FRUITS AND VEGETABLES

23

Breads

WHOLE-WHEAT FRENCH BREAD

The only difference between this and white French bread is the extra fiber in the whole-wheat version.

Makes 4 loaves — 12 slices each loaf

1 tablespoon active dry yeast
1 tablespoon sugar
1 teaspoon salt
2½ cups lukewarm water
3 cups whole-wheat flour

2–3 cups unbleached white
  flour
1 egg white mixed with 1
  tablespoon cold water

Combine yeast, sugar, salt, and water in a large bowl. Gradually add flours and mix well. Dough may be very sticky; add enough flour to transfer it to a lightly floured board. Knead about 10 minutes, adding more flour as necessary to keep it from sticking.

Place dough in bowl lightly sprayed with nonstick cooking spray. Cover with damp cloth; let rise in warm place until it doubles in size, 1½–2 hours. Punch dough down.

Transfer dough to floured board and cut into 4 equal pieces. Roll and shape each piece into a long loaf. Place loaves in baguette pans sprayed with nonstick cooking spray. Slash top of each loaf in three or four places and brush with egg white and water. Let dough rise another hour or until doubled in volume.

Heat oven to 350 degrees. Bake loaves until browned and hollow-sounding when tapped, about 25 minutes. Halfway through baking, it may be necessary to cover loaves with aluminum foil to prevent tops from scorching. Remove from pans and cool on racks.

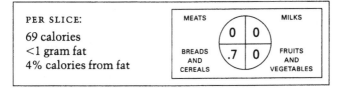

PER SLICE:
69 calories
<1 gram fat
4% calories from fat

MEATS 0   MILKS 0
BREADS AND CEREALS .7   FRUITS AND VEGETABLES 0

DILL BREAD

My daughter accused me of cheating when I used packaged hot-roll mix in this recipe. I think it's a clever shortcut.

Makes 1 loaf

1 package hot-roll mix
1 tablespoon dried dill
¾ cup very hot water (120–130 degrees F)
½ cup nonfat small-curd cottage cheese

2 tablespoons oil
2 egg whites
1 tablespoon melted reduced-calorie margarine

In large bowl, combine roll mix with yeast from foil packet and dill; mix well. Stir in hot water, cottage cheese, oil, and egg whites and mix until dough pulls away from sides of bowl. Turn dough out onto lightly floured surface. With greased or floured hands, shape dough into a ball. Knead 5 minutes or until smooth. Cover with large bowl and let rest 5 minutes.

Grease 8-inch round cake pan and press dough onto bottom. Cover dough and let rise in warm place 30 minutes or until doubled in size.

Heat oven to 350 degrees. Uncover dough. Bake 40–50 minutes or until golden brown and loaf sounds hollow when lightly tapped. Remove loaf from pan and brush top with margarine. Cool on wire rack.

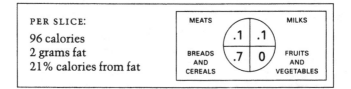

PER SLICE:
96 calories
2 grams fat
21% calories from fat

MEATS .1 | .1 MILKS
BREADS AND CEREALS .7 | 0 FRUITS AND VEGETABLES

YOGURT SOURDOUGH BREAD

Makes 2 loaves — 12 slices each loaf

6 cups flour
2 packages active dry yeast
2 tablespoons sugar
1½ teaspoons salt
1 cup nonfat plain yogurt at
  room temperature

1 cup water
1 tablespoon shortening,
  softened
1 tablespoon nonfat milk

In a large bowl, mix 2 cups flour, yeast, sugar, and salt. Put yogurt in small bowl and add water, stirring until well blended; add shortening and continue to stir. Add yogurt mixture to flour mixture. Using an electric mixer, beat at low speed until all ingredients are well blended. Increase speed to medium and stir in as much flour as it takes to make a firm dough. Knead dough on lightly floured surface until smooth and elastic, 5–10 minutes.

Spray another bowl with nonstick cooking spray; place dough in bowl and turn to coat with spray; cover and let rise in a warm place about 1 hour or until doubled in bulk. Punch dough down, cover, and let rise again until doubled in bulk. Punch dough down again and divide in half. On a lightly floured surface, roll each piece of dough out to a 6 × 12-inch rectangle.

Starting with the short side, roll dough up tightly like a jelly roll; pinch edges to seal. Place each piece in a nonstick loaf pan sprayed with nonstick cooking spray. Let rise until doubled again. Brush top with milk.

Bake at 400 degrees until golden brown, about 35 minutes. Remove from pans and cool on wire rack.

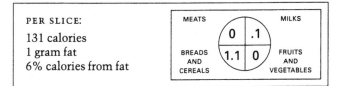

PER SLICE:		
131 calories		
1 gram fat		
6% calories from fat		

	MEATS	MILKS
	0	.1
	BREADS AND CEREALS	FRUITS AND VEGETABLES
	1.1	0

HERB DINNER ROLLS

If you were to lather one of these rolls with butter, you'd convert it to 43 percent fat calories!

Makes 16 rolls

1 package hot-roll mix
1 cup very hot water (120–130 degrees F)
2 tablespoons reduced-calorie margarine, softened
2 egg whites

1 tablespoon dried parsley
3 tablespoons dried basil
2 teaspoons dried thyme
1 tablespoon melted reduced-calorie margarine (optional)

In large bowl, combine roll mix with yeast from foil packet; blend well. Add hot water, margarine, egg whites, parsley, basil, and thyme and stir until dough pulls away from sides of bowl. Turn dough out onto lightly floured surface. With greased or floured hands, shape dough into a ball. Knead 5 minutes or until smooth and cover with large bowl. Let rest 5 minutes.

Spray two cookie sheets with nonstick cooking spray. Divide dough in half; cut each half into 8 pieces. Shape each piece into a ball. Place 8 balls on each spray-coated cookie sheet. Cover with lightweight towel; let rise in warm place 30 minutes or until doubled in size.

Heat oven to 350 degrees. Uncover dough. Bake rolls 15–20 minutes or until light golden brown. Brush tops with melted margarine if desired. Serve warm.

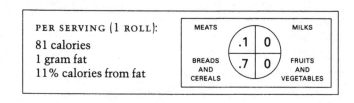

PER SERVING (1 ROLL):
81 calories
1 gram fat
11% calories from fat

	MEATS	MILKS
	.1	0
BREADS AND CEREALS	.7	0 FRUITS AND VEGETABLES

LITE BREAKFAST ROLLS

Makes 18 rolls

ROLLS

1 package hot-roll mix
1 cup very hot water (120 to
   130 degrees F)
2 tablespoons reduced-calorie
   margarine, softened

2 egg whites
2 tablespoons apple juice
⅓ cup firmly packed brown
   sugar
2 teaspoons cinnamon

GLAZE

¼ cup powdered sugar   2–3 teaspoons nonfat milk

In large bowl, combine roll mix with yeast from foil packet; blend well. Stir in hot water, margarine, and egg whites until dough pulls away from sides of bowl. Turn dough out onto lightly floured surface. With greased or floured hands, shape dough into a ball. Knead dough 5 minutes or until smooth. Cover dough with large bowl. Let rest 5 minutes.

Spray two 8- or 9-inch square pans with nonstick cooking spray. On lightly floured surface, roll dough to 18 × 10-inch rectangle. Brush with apple juice. In small bowl, combine brown sugar and cinnamon; mix well. Sprinkle evenly over dough. Starting with 18-inch side, roll up tightly, pressing edge to seal. Cut into 18 slices. Place cut side down in spray-coated pans. Cover with lightweight towel; let rise in warm place 30 minutes or until doubled in size.

Heat oven to 375 degrees. Uncover rolls. Bake 20–25 minutes or until golden brown. In small bowl, combine powdered sugar and enough milk for desired glaze consistency. Blend until smooth. Drizzle over warm rolls.

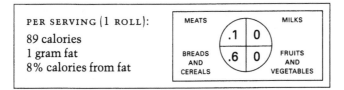

PER SERVING (1 ROLL):
89 calories
1 gram fat
8% calories from fat

	MEATS		MILKS
		.1	0
	BREADS AND CEREALS	.6	0 FRUITS AND VEGETABLES

BOSTON BROWN BREAD

This is good enough for dessert!

Makes 1 loaf — 12 slices

1 cup whole-wheat flour
1 cup rye flour
1 cup whole cornmeal
¾ teaspoon baking soda
1 teaspoon salt

2 cups buttermilk (or 1 cup
plain yogurt mixed with 1
cup nonfat milk)
¾ cup molasses
1 cup raisins

Combine dry ingredients in one bowl and wet ingredients and raisins in another bowl, then mix the two together. Pour into 3-pound coffee can sprayed with nonstick cooking spray. Mixture should fill can ¾ full. Cover can with waxed paper, foil, or paper and tie with a string. Place can in a big stewpot. Pour hot water into pot to ¾ height of can. Cover pot. Bring water to boil and steam on top of stove 2½ hours.

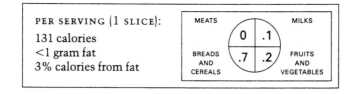

PER SERVING (1 SLICE):
131 calories
<1 gram fat
3% calories from fat

MEATS   MILKS
0   .1
BREADS AND CEREALS   .7   .2   FRUITS AND VEGETABLES

*I*ncrease the fiber in bread recipes by substituting 1 cup less two tablespoons of whole-grain flour for each cup of white flour. As the amount of white flour decreases, the bread becomes heavier and coarser. Bread that is 100 percent whole-wheat is delicious but rather solid! You may prefer half to two-thirds white flour.

EASY APPLESAUCE MUFFINS

Makes 12 muffins

2 cups regular Cheerios cereal,
  crushed
1¼ cups unbleached white
  flour
⅓ cup packed brown sugar
2 teaspoons ground cinnamon
1¼ teaspoons baking powder

¾ teaspoon baking soda
2 tablespoons safflower oil
⅓ cup nonfat milk
1 cup unsweetened applesauce
½ cup raisins
1 egg white

Heat oven to 400 degrees. Mix dry ingredients in a large bowl. Combine remaining ingredients and stir into dry ingredients until moistened. Divide batter evenly in a nonstick muffin pan. Bake until golden brown, 18–22 minutes.

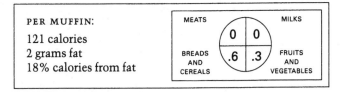

PER MUFFIN:

121 calories
2 grams fat
18% calories from fat

MEATS 0 | MILKS 0
BREADS AND CEREALS .6 | FRUITS AND VEGETABLES .3

*C*onsider adding ¼ cup of 100 percent bran, wheat germ, or cracked wheat to your bread recipe. This will add fiber and nourishment to the finished product without changing the taste.

OATMEAL MUFFINS

I wrap leftover muffins individually in plastic wrap and freeze them. Then I can eat one or two with several meals to come.

Makes 12 muffins

1¼ cups white flour
1 cup rolled oats
½ cup raisins
¼ cup brown sugar
1 tablespoon baking powder

¾ teaspoon cinnamon
½ teaspoon salt
1 egg, slightly beaten
1 cup nonfat milk
¼ cup oil

Heat oven to 400 degrees. Combine flour, oats, raisins, brown sugar, baking powder, cinnamon, and salt; set aside. In a small bowl, mix egg, milk, and oil. Pour into flour mixture and stir until moistened. Pour into nonstick muffin cups. Bake at 400 degrees for 20 minutes or until toothpick inserted in center of muffin comes out clean.

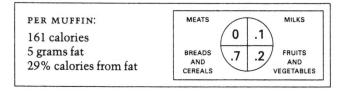

PER MUFFIN:
161 calories
5 grams fat
29% calories from fat

MEATS 0 | .1 MILKS
BREADS AND CEREALS .7 | .2 FRUITS AND VEGETABLES

CINNAMON-APPLE SCONES

In the original recipe, each scone had 6 grams of fat.

Makes 12 scones

½ cup unbleached flour
½ cup whole-wheat flour
1½ teaspoons baking powder
½ teaspoon ground cinnamon
1 tablespoon margarine
1 small apple, peeled and cored
1 cup quick-cooking rolled oats

2 egg whites
2 tablespoons apple juice or
    nonfat milk
⅓ cup low-fat or nonfat
    buttermilk
2 tablespoons honey
nonfat milk

Heat oven to 400 degrees. In a bowl, combine flours, baking powder, and cinnamon. Cut in margarine until mixture resembles coarse crumbs. Chop apple into small pieces; mix with oats into flour mixture. Add egg whites, apple juice or milk, buttermilk, and honey; mix well (dough will be sticky). Spray baking sheet with nonstick cooking spray. With floured hands, pat dough into 7-inch circle on baking sheet. Cut into 12 equal wedges; using a spatula with a long thin blade, separate wedges 1 inch apart. Brush with milk. Bake 10–12 minutes or until golden brown.

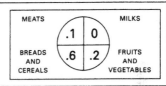

PER SCONE:

102 calories
2 grams fat
16% calories from fat

OAT-BRAN MUFFINS

A fast-food bran muffin has 6 grams of fat.

Makes 12 muffins

1¼ cups oat bran
1 cup unbleached white flour
1 1-ounce packet instant plain
*   oatmeal*
¾ cup raisins (optional)
1 tablespoon baking powder

1 teaspoon cinnamon
½ teaspoon allspice
1¾ cups nonfat milk
3 egg whites, beaten
1 tablespoon safflower oil

Heat oven to 425 degrees. Mix all of the above ingredients together and pour into muffin tins lightly coated with nonstick cooking spray. Bake 15–17 minutes or until tops are golden brown.

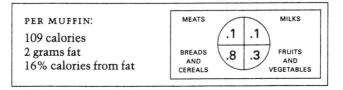

PER MUFFIN:

109 calories
2 grams fat
16% calories from fat

SUMMER-BERRY BUTTERMILK PANCAKES

In Oregon we love to use marionberries or raspberries, but any berry will work.

Makes 12 pancakes

1 cup low-fat buttermilk	1 tablespoon sugar
1 egg	1 teaspoon baking powder
1 egg white	1/2 teaspoon baking soda
1 tablespoon oil	1/2 teaspoon salt
1 cup white flour	1 cup berries, fresh or frozen

Beat together buttermilk, egg, egg white, and oil. Mix dry ingredients together and add to liquid mixture, blending well. Stir berries in gently (if frozen, no need to thaw). Heat nonstick frying pan medium-hot. Brown pancakes on both sides until firm to touch.

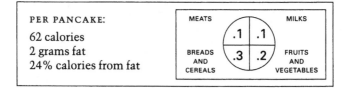

PER PANCAKE:

62 calories
2 grams fat
24% calories from fat

MEATS .1 | MILKS .1
BREADS AND CEREALS .3 | FRUITS AND VEGETABLES .2

These days waffles and pancakes are usually relegated to weekend breakfasts. That's too bad — with prepared low-fat mixes and a nonstick griddle or waffle iron, you can have delicious pancakes and waffles in just five minutes. And you can add a variety of ingredients from the milk and fruits and vegetables groups.

24

Desserts

The recipes in this section are all low in fat, *but* some of them contain sugar. So a word of caution — you may eat from this section **if** you have exercised today.

APPLE CRISP

The oatmeal in this dessert gives you apple-pie satisfaction without the fat.

Serves 6

4 cups tart apples, peeled and
   sliced
¼ cup instant oatmeal
¼ cup unbleached white flour
⅓ cup brown sugar

½ teaspoon cinnamon
¼ teaspoon nutmeg
1½ tablespoons margarine,
   softened

Heat oven to 375 degrees. Spray 8-inch-square baking pan with nonstick cooking spray. Spread apple slices to cover pan. Mix remaining ingredients thoroughly. Sprinkle over apples. Bake at 375 degrees for 30 minutes or until apples are tender and topping is golden brown. Serve warm with nonfat vanilla yogurt or frozen yogurt if desired.

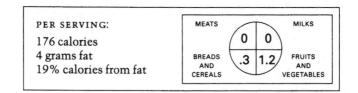

PER SERVING:
176 calories
4 grams fat
19% calories from fat

MEATS 0 | MILKS 0
BREADS AND CEREALS .3 | 1.2 FRUITS AND VEGETABLES

CREAMY FRUIT TACOS

Combining fruit and salty tacos sounds strange, but it's delicious.

Serves 8

*2 8-ounce packages nonfat
  cream cheese, softened*
1 tablespoon grated orange rind
*2 tablespoons sugar or one
  package sugar substitute*
3 tablespoons orange juice
*2 oranges, peeled and cut into
  pieces*

1 cup sliced strawberries
1 kiwi, peeled and sliced
1 banana, peeled and sliced
*1 cup canned pineapple
  chunks, drained*
1 box taco shells

In medium-sized bowl, blend cream cheese with orange rind, sugar, and orange juice; chill. In large bowl, combine fruits; chill. Heat taco shells in oven until warm. Spread cream cheese mixture in shells; top with fruit. Serve immediately.

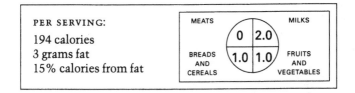

PER SERVING:
194 calories
3 grams fat
15% calories from fat

	MEATS		MILKS
	0	2.0	
BREADS AND CEREALS	1.0	1.0	FRUITS AND VEGETABLES

DELECTABLE FRUIT

Serves 12

1 20-ounce can pineapple
    chunks
2 11-ounce cans mandarin
    oranges
1 cup red seedless grapes

2 kiwis, halved lengthwise,
    peeled, and sliced
$\frac{1}{2}$ cup orange juice
$\frac{1}{4}$ cup honey
1 tablespoon lemon juice

Drain pineapple and mandarin oranges; reserve juice. In large bowl, combine pineapple, mandarin oranges, grapes, and kiwi. Mix reserved juices, orange juice, honey, and lemon juice. Pour over fruit. Cover and chill until ready to serve.

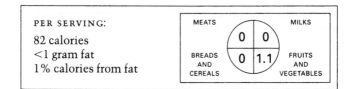

PER SERVING:
82 calories
<1 gram fat
1% calories from fat

MEATS   MILKS
0   0
BREADS AND CEREALS   0   1.1   FRUITS AND VEGETABLES

FRUIT COMBO

Serves 10

2 cups pitted sweet cherries
$\frac{1}{2}$ honeydew melon, cubed

$\frac{1}{2}$ cantaloupe, sliced and cubed
1 orange, peeled and sectioned

Combine ingredients and chill. If desired, top with Autumn Fruit Dressing.

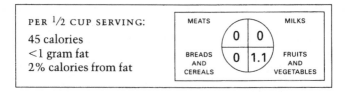

PER $\frac{1}{2}$ CUP SERVING:
45 calories
<1 gram fat
2% calories from fat

MEATS   MILKS
0   0
BREADS AND CEREALS   0   1.1   FRUITS AND VEGETABLES

AUTUMN FRUIT DRESSING

Makes 1 cup

This is also good over frozen vanilla yogurt.

½ cup apple juice
½ cup orange juice
2 tablespoons brown sugar
¼ teaspoon nutmeg

¼ teaspoon allspice
1 cinnamon stick or 1 teaspoon
  ground cinnamon

Combine all ingredients in saucepan and bring to a boil. Reduce heat and simmer for about 5 minutes or until thick. Cool and use over fruit.

PER TABLESPOON:		MEATS			MILKS
14 calories			0	0	
<1 gram fat		BREADS AND CEREALS	0	.1	FRUITS AND VEGETABLES
3% calories from fat					

RAINBOW FRUIT

Serves 12

2 cups watermelon cubes
2 cups cantaloupe cubes
2 cups green grapes

2 cups hulled strawberries
2 cups fresh blueberries

Combine all fruits in large bowl. Toss gently; cover and chill if desired. Serve with Orange-Marshmallow Dressing.

PER SERVING:		MEATS			MILKS
45 calories			0	0	
<1 gram fat		BREADS AND CEREALS	0	1.7	FRUITS AND VEGETABLES
2% calories from fat					

ORANGE-MARSHMALLOW DRESSING

I also spread this on graham crackers for a sweet snack.

1 cup nonfat cream cheese   *1 teaspoon grated orange rind*
1 cup marshmallow spread

Combine ingredients in a bowl and blend thoroughly.

PER TABLESPOON:		MEATS		MILKS
18 calories		0	.3	
<1 gram fat		BREADS AND CEREALS	0	0	FRUITS AND VEGETABLES
0% calories from fat				

PEACH MELBA MOLD

Use any fruit that's plentiful. Kids love this dessert.

Serves 8

1 3-ounce package   *1 3-ounce package*
  raspberry-flavored gelatin   *peach-flavored gelatin*
1¾ cup boiling water, divided   *2 cups peeled, sliced peaches*
1 cup cold water   *2 tablespoons lemon juice*
1 cup raspberries   *1 cup whipped low-fat topping*

In medium-sized bowl, dissolve raspberry gelatin in 1 cup boiling water; stir in cold water. Refrigerate until thickened but not set, 30–40 minutes. Lightly oil a 6-cup mold, or spray with nonstick cooking spray. Stir raspberries into thickened gelatin. Pour into oiled mold. Refrigerate until firm, about 30 minutes.

Meanwhile, dissolve peach gelatin in ¾ cup boiling water; cool. Put peaches and lemon juice into blender; blend until smooth. Add 1¼ cups puréed mixture (if necessary, add water to make this amount) to peach gelatin. Refrigerate until thickened but not set, about 30 minutes. Fold in whipped topping. Spoon peach mixture evenly over raspberry mixture in mold. Refrigerate until firm. To serve, unmold onto serving plate.

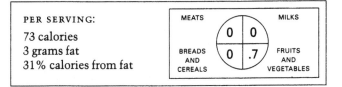

PER SERVING:
73 calories
3 grams fat
31% calories from fat

MEATS 0 0 MILKS
BREADS AND CEREALS 0 .7 FRUITS AND VEGETABLES

PEACH MERINGUE TARTS

Once you get the hang of making nonfat meringue cups, you'll use them all the time.

Serves 6

2 egg whites
1/8 teaspoon cream of tartar
1/8 teaspoon nutmeg
2/3 cup granulated sugar
1 6-ounce can frozen cranberry juice concentrate

1/2 cup water
1 1/2 tablespoons cornstarch
3 cups sliced peaches, fresh or canned

Heat oven to 150 degrees. Place egg whites in mixing bowl, add cream of tartar and nutmeg, and beat until foamy. Gradually add sugar, beating constantly, until meringue is stiff. Divide into 6 mounds on nonstick baking sheet. With back of spoon, shape into round tart shells. Bake at 150 degrees for 1 hour. Cool. Thaw cranberry juice concentrate and pour into saucepan. Mix water and cornstarch until smooth and stir into concentrate. Cook, stirring constantly, until sauce thickens and is clear; cool. Fill each meringue tart with 1/2 cup peach slices. Spoon sauce over fruit.

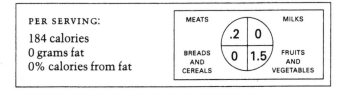

PER SERVING:
184 calories
0 grams fat
0% calories from fat

MEATS .2 0 MILKS
BREADS AND CEREALS 0 1.5 FRUITS AND VEGETABLES

PUMPKIN PUDDING "PIE"

You can use 2 cups of mashed fresh pumpkin instead of canned pumpkin.

Serves 4

1 12-ounce can pumpkin	*2 teaspoons pumpkin pie spice*
1 12-ounce can evaporated	*1 whole egg*
skim milk	*⅓ cup honey*
2 egg whites	

Heat oven to 350 degrees. Put all ingredients in a bowl and mix well. Spray 9-inch pie plate with nonstick cooking spray and pour mixture into pie plate. Bake at 350 degrees 45 minutes.

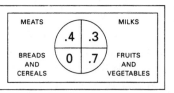

PER SERVING:
187 calories
2 grams fat
8% calories from fat

MEATS .4 | .3 MILKS
BREADS AND CEREALS 0 | .7 FRUITS AND VEGETABLES

STRAWBERRY CREAM CHEESE PIE

There's fat in this pie crust because I've never found a satisfying fat-free "crust." The filling has no fat, however, so the finished product is only 26 percent fat.

Serves 6

CRUST

1 cup crushed graham cracker	*2 tablespoons melted butter*
crumbs	

Mix together crumbs and butter until evenly moistened. Pat into 7-inch pie plate and bake at 350 degrees 10 minutes. Let cool.

FILLING

1 envelope gelatin	3 egg whites
¼ cup water	¼ cup evaporated skim milk,
¾ cup nonfat cottage cheese	chilled very cold
4 ounces nonfat cream cheese	2 tablespoons sugar
2 cups crushed strawberries	

Soften gelatin in water, then bring to a boil to dissolve. Blend cottage cheese with cream cheese in food processor until smooth. Beat together gelatin, cottage cheese/cream cheese mixture, and crushed berries.

In separate bowl, beat egg whites until stiff. In another bowl, whip evaporated skim milk until peaks form, then stir in sugar. Gently fold together egg whites and whipped milk, then fold this mixture carefully into the berry mixture. Pour gently into cooled pie shell and refrigerate until firm.

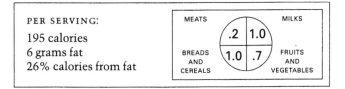

PER SERVING:
195 calories
6 grams fat
26% calories from fat

MEATS .2 | MILKS 1.0
BREADS AND CEREALS 1.0 | FRUITS AND VEGETABLES .7

STRAWBERRY DUMPLINGS

The berries in this recipe create the sauce for the dumplings. I like strawberries, but blackberries or raspberries work equally well.

Serves 6

4½ cups strawberries	1½ teaspoons baking powder
½ cup plus 2 tablespoons sugar	½ teaspoon salt
¼ cup water	½ cup nonfat milk
1 cup unbleached white flour	1½ tablespoons oil

Combine berries, ½ cup sugar, and water in 2-quart casserole dish. Microwave on high for 5 minutes or until mixture starts to boil.

Combine flour, 2 tablespoons sugar, baking powder, and salt. In separate bowl, combine milk and oil. Add to dry ingredients. Stir just until mixed, with no dry ingredients showing. Do not overmix! Drop by spoonfuls onto hot fruit mixture. Cover with tight-fitting lid. Microwave on high for 5 minutes or until dumplings are no longer doughy. You will see them rise and fluff up. Do not remove lid until you're sure they are done. Serve with ice milk or low-fat frozen yogurt.

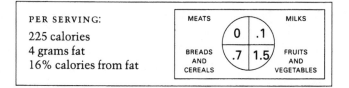

PER SERVING:
225 calories
4 grams fat
16% calories from fat

MEATS			MILKS
	0	.1	
BREADS AND CEREALS	.7	1.5	FRUITS AND VEGETABLES

ANY-BERRY PAVLOVA

This is my favorite frozen dessert. For an even "richer" dessert (but no extra fat), spread a layer of softened nonfat cream cheese over the yogurt.

Serves 9

3 egg whites
1/8 teaspoon salt
1/8 teaspoon cream of tartar
1/3 cup sugar

1/2 teaspoon vanilla
1 cup nonfat vanilla yogurt
4 cups fresh berries, washed
*   and sliced*

Heat oven to 450 degrees. Beat egg whites until foamy and add salt and cream of tartar. Beat again until very stiff; add sugar and vanilla. Spread meringue in an 8-inch-square baking dish; place in oven and turn off heat immediately; leave in oven without opening door for 8 hours or overnight.

Stir yogurt until smooth, spread on top of meringue, and cover with plastic wrap. Freeze 4–6 hours or until firm. Cover with fresh berries and cut into squares to serve.

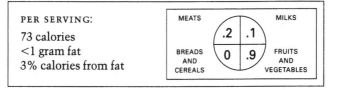

PER SERVING:
73 calories
<1 gram fat
3% calories from fat

MEATS .2 | .1 MILKS
BREADS AND CEREALS 0 | .9 FRUITS AND VEGETABLES

TANTALIZING TRIFLE

Angel-food cake is a bargain because it contains NO fat. And if you use nonfat ricotta cheese, there will be no fat in the recipe.

Serves 4

⅙ angel-food cake or
  4 × 5-inch piece
2 tablespoons orange liqueur
½ cup canned water-packed
  peaches, drained

2 tablespoons cornstarch
3 tablespoons sugar, divided
1½ cups nonfat milk
1 teaspoon vanilla
½ cup low-fat ricotta cheese

Cut cake into 1-inch cubes. Press into bottom of shallow 1-quart bowl; sprinkle with orange liqueur, then layer peaches over top.

Prepare sauce by mixing together cornstarch and 2 tablespoons sugar and adding milk. Bring to a boil, stirring constantly, and cook 1 minute or until thick. Add vanilla.

Beat ricotta cheese and 1 tablespoon sugar until smooth; stir into sauce. Pour sauce over soaked cake and let stand in refrigerator several hours or overnight for flavors to blend.

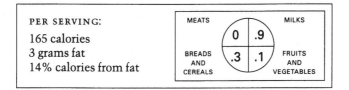

PER SERVING:
165 calories
3 grams fat
14% calories from fat

MEATS 0 | .9 MILKS
BREADS AND CEREALS .3 | .1 FRUITS AND VEGETABLES

BANANA-BERRY SHERBET

The lemon juice keeps the bananas from turning brown and gives the sherbet a flavorful lift.

Serves 6

*1 large ripe banana, cut into
    ¼-inch slices
2 teaspoons lemon juice*

*⅔ cup unsweetened frozen
    strawberries, unthawed
½ cup unsweetened apple
    juice, chilled*

Combine banana slices and lemon juice in small bowl. Arrange in single layer on baking sheet or in plastic sandwich bags; cover and freeze until firm. Place bananas and strawberries in food processor; process until finely chopped. Add apple juice and process until smooth; scrape sides of bowl occasionally, using rubber spatula. Serve immediately or spoon into serving dishes and freeze up to 1 hour.

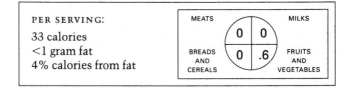

PER SERVING:		
33 calories	MEATS 0	MILKS 0
<1 gram fat	BREADS AND CEREALS 0	FRUITS AND VEGETABLES .6
4% calories from fat		

*H*ave some old bananas on hand? Freeze them and mix with the flavored yogurt of your choice. Add a dash of vanilla and purée in the blender. You will have a delicious dessert.

FRUIT AND YOGURT CRUNCH POPS

Kids love the crunchy texture of these nutritious frozen popsicles. You can mix and match various kinds of yogurt and fruit.

Serves 8

1 cup nonfat vanilla frozen yogurt	*¼ cup low-fat granola cereal, crushed*
1 cup mashed strawberries	*8 3-ounce cold-drink cups*
1 tablespoon honey (optional)	*8 wooden sticks*

In medium-sized bowl, combine frozen yogurt, strawberries, and honey; mix well. Place about 1 teaspoon crushed cereal in bottom of each cup and spoon in scant ¼ cup yogurt mixture. Insert stick into center of mixture. Freeze 3–4 hours or until firm. To serve, remove drink cups.

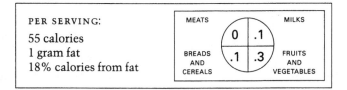

PER SERVING:
55 calories
1 gram fat
18% calories from fat

MEATS 0
MILKS .1
BREADS AND CEREALS .1
FRUITS AND VEGETABLES .3

LIME-MINT ICE

Here's a super-simple but elegant way to use leftover champagne.

Serves 8

⅔ cup sugar	*4–5 limes, cut in half lengthwise*
½ cup water	*1 cup champagne or white wine*
30 fresh mint leaves	

Bring sugar and water to boil over medium-high heat in nonaluminum saucepan. Remove from heat and add mint leaves. Steep for five minutes. Squeeze enough lime juice to measure ⅔ cup; save limes and pulp. Strain out any seeds from juice; add juice and champagne or wine to mint syrup and stir. Remove mint leaves and pour mixture into cold glass bowl; place in freezer for 6 hours or until frozen; stir mixture occasionally. Meanwhile, cut thin slice of rind from outer curve of each lime half so it will sit flat; using paring knife, remove remaining pulp from rind.

Remove ice from freezer about 30 minutes before serving. When ice softens, scoop into lime shells. Return to freezer until ready to serve. Garnish with mint. If desired, drizzle melted chocolate over top.

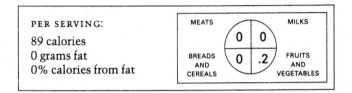

PER SERVING:
89 calories
0 grams fat
0% calories from fat

	MEATS	MILKS
	0	0
	BREADS AND CEREALS	FRUITS AND VEGETABLES
	0	.2

FRUIT ICES

You can quickly prepare frozen treats in a variety of ways for scrumptious snacks or summer desserts. Here are a few suggestions.

Each recipe serves 8

PINEAPPLE ICE

2 cups pineapple   *1 tablespoon sugar*
2 tablespoons lemon juice

KIWI ICE

12 kiwis   *2 tablespoons lemon juice*
2 tablespoons lime juice   *2 tablespoons sugar*

MELON ICE

*4 cups watermelon, seeds   *2 tablespoons lemon juice*
   removed*   *2 tablespoons sugar*

Put fruit in food processor and purée thoroughly; add lemon juice and sugar. Pour into ice-cube tray for freezing. When almost frozen, return to food processor and purée again. Repeat the purée/freeze process at least one more time (to prevent crystals from forming). Serve and enjoy!

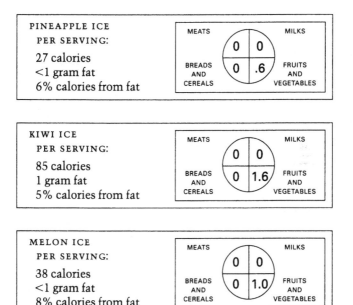

PINEAPPLE ICE
PER SERVING:
27 calories
<1 gram fat
6% calories from fat

MEATS 0 | MILKS 0
BREADS AND CEREALS 0 | FRUITS AND VEGETABLES .6

KIWI ICE
PER SERVING:
85 calories
1 gram fat
5% calories from fat

MEATS 0 | MILKS 0
BREADS AND CEREALS 0 | FRUITS AND VEGETABLES 1.6

MELON ICE
PER SERVING:
38 calories
<1 gram fat
8% calories from fat

MEATS 0 | MILKS 0
BREADS AND CEREALS 0 | FRUITS AND VEGETABLES 1.0

ORANGE-PEACH SORBET

Fruit gets sweeter as it ripens. If you use very ripe fruit you can omit the sugar.

Serves 6

6 peaches, sliced
3 tablespoons sugar

1 cup orange juice
1 teaspoon Tang powder

Place all ingredients in blender and purée. Pour into loaf pan and freeze. Place in blender again and whip. Pour into pan and freeze a second time.

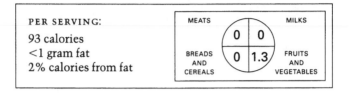

PER SERVING:		
93 calories	MEATS **0**	MILKS **0**
<1 gram fat	BREADS AND CEREALS **0**	FRUITS AND VEGETABLES **1.3**
2% calories from fat		

LOW-FAT BAKED ALASKA

For an elegant presentation, serve this on a glass cake plate. Make sure the plate will tolerate a hot oven for one minute when you brown the meringue.

Serves 12

1 pint chocolate nonfat frozen yogurt, slightly softened
1 pint strawberry nonfat frozen yogurt, slightly softened
1 8-inch angel-food cake, cut in two layers

5 egg whites at room temperature
½ teaspoon cream of tartar
½ teaspoon vanilla extract
¼ cup sugar

Line two 8-inch cake pans with wax paper, leaving an overhang around the edges. Spread chocolate frozen yogurt evenly into one pan and strawberry frozen yogurt into the other; freeze until each is firm. Place one cake layer on a serving dish. Invert chocolate yogurt onto the cake, then invert strawberry layer onto the chocolate. Cover with second cake layer and place in freezer until frozen yogurt is firm.

Heat oven to 475 degrees. Beat egg whites until foamy, add cream of tartar and vanilla, and beat until soft peaks form. Gradually add sugar, 1 tablespoon at a time, and beat until stiff peaks form. Remove cake from freezer and quickly spread meringue over entire surface, making sure edges are sealed to serving plate. Bake at 475 degrees 1 minute or until meringue peaks are lightly browned. Slice into wedges and serve immediately.

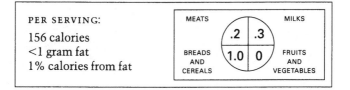

LOW-FAT ICE CREAM BALLS

I sometimes use butterscotch pudding for a very different taste.

Serves 8

*1 quart nonfat vanilla or
   chocolate frozen yogurt*
*1 package sugar-free Jell-O
   chocolate pudding*

1 cup evaporated skim milk
1 cup water

Allow frozen yogurt to soften slightly. Mix chocolate pudding with evaporated skim milk and water; beat well. Using an ice cream scoop, form frozen yogurt into balls (approximately 6). Place on a platter and lightly ice with chocolate pudding. Put in freezer. (Don't put too much pudding on the ice cream balls, or they will be hard to eat.) When frozen solid, serve.

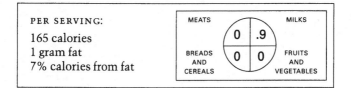

When fit people eat sugar, they store it in their muscles for tomorrow's run. When fat people eat sugar, they store it in their fat cells.

CHEESECAKE

Serves 12

1¼ cup graham cracker crumbs   5 egg whites
¼ cup melted margarine   1 pint nonfat vanilla yogurt
8 ounces low-fat cream cheese   1 teaspoon vanilla
½ cup sugar

Heat oven to 350 degrees. Mix crumbs and margarine; press into bottom and sides of 9-inch pie plate. Mix cream cheese, sugar, and egg whites in blender or food processor until smooth; pour into crust. Bake at 350 degrees for 20 minutes. Cool. Mix together vanilla and yogurt; pour over cooked cream cheese mixture. Bake at 350 degrees for another 20 minutes. Chill well before serving.

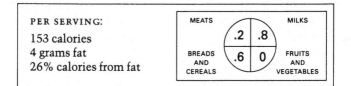

PER SERVING:
153 calories
4 grams fat
26% calories from fat

MEATS .2 | .8 MILKS
BREADS AND CEREALS .6 | 0 FRUITS AND VEGETABLES

I never make a New Year's resolution to exercise! For me, exercise is like brushing my teeth or putting on clothes in the morning. I don't have to resolve to do something that is an important part of my lifestyle. I may occasionally skip for a day or two, but I know I'll go back to it.

CRUSTLESS CHEESECAKE

Your guests will cheer these lower-in-fat versions of traditional cheesecakes. They're delicious plain and superb when topped with glazed fruit.

Serves 12

4 cups nonfat or low-fat ricotta
  cheese
2 egg yolks
1 cup nonfat buttermilk
½ cup (or less) sugar
1 tablespoon cornstarch

2 teaspoons vanilla extract
¼ teaspoon salt
juice of one small lemon
1 tablespoon grated lemon rind
5 egg whites

Heat oven to 375 degrees. In large bowl, beat ricotta cheese until smooth. Add egg yolks one at a time, beating well after each addition; add buttermilk, sugar, cornstarch, vanilla, salt, lemon juice, and lemon rind. Slowly pour in egg whites and beat until mixture is thick. Pour batter into 9-inch springform pan sprayed with nonstick cooking spray. Bake at 375 degrees for 1 hour.

Cool completely before serving. If desired, garnish with fresh fruit or fruit-flavored yogurt or frost with flavored yogurt cheese.

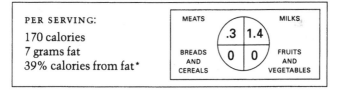

PER SERVING:		
170 calories	MEATS .3	MILKS 1.4
7 grams fat	BREADS AND CEREALS 0	FRUITS AND VEGETABLES 0
39% calories from fat*		

To release more juice from lemons, let them come to room temperature before cutting and squeezing, or microwave for one minute on medium power.

* See p. 47, no. 1.

KISSES

You can add chopped nuts or coconut to these cookies, but they will be higher in fat.

Makes about 16

4 egg whites   1 teaspoon vanilla
1¼ cups powdered sugar

Heat oven to 225 degrees. Beat egg whites until stiff and gradually add ⅔ cup sugar. Continue beating until mixture is stiff and holds its shape. Fold in remaining sugar and vanilla. Drop mixture from tip of spoon in small (tablespoon-size) piles ½ inch apart on nonstick pan. Bake at 225 degrees until very light brown, about 4 minutes.

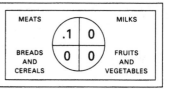

PER KISS:

35 calories
0 grams fat
0% calories from fat

	MEATS	MILKS
	.1	0
BREADS AND CEREALS	0	0
		FRUITS AND VEGETABLES

COCOA MERINGUE COOKIES

I can eat a dozen of these and not feel guilty!

Makes 30

3 egg whites   3 tablespoons unsweetened
¼ teaspoon cream of tartar   baking cocoa
½ cup sugar, divided   1 tablespoon cornstarch

Heat oven to 325 degrees. Place rack in upper third of oven. Beat egg whites until foamy, add cream of tartar, and beat until mixture forms soft peaks. Add ¼ cup sugar and continue beating until stiff. In separate bowl, mix ¼ cup sugar, cocoa, and cornstarch. Fold into meringue. Cover cookie sheet with foil and spray with nonstick cooking spray. Drop meringue onto foil by tablespoons. Bake for 30 minutes or until set. Do not overbake.

PER COOKIE:		
6 calories		
<1 gram fat		
4% calories from fat		

	MEATS	MILKS
	0	0
BREADS AND CEREALS	0	0	FRUITS AND VEGETABLES

COFFEE MERINGUE COOKIES

You'll love this adaptation of the traditional meringue recipe.

Makes 30

3 egg whites	*¾ teaspoon instant coffee*
⅛ teaspoon salt	* powder*
½ teaspoon cream of tartar	*dash of nutmeg*
¾ cup sugar	*¼ teaspoon grated lemon peel*
	1 teaspoon vanilla

Heat oven to 350 degrees. Beat egg whites until fluffy. Add salt and cream of tartar and continue beating. Add sugar slowly, beating constantly, until meringue is glossy. Place half the meringue in separate bowl and fold in coffee powder, nutmeg, lemon peel, and vanilla. Fold in remaining meringue. Drop by tablespoons onto baking sheet. Put in preheated oven. Turn off oven immediately and leave cookies in oven until cooled, at least 2 hours.

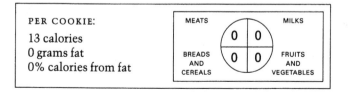

PER COOKIE:		
13 calories		
0 grams fat		
0% calories from fat		

	MEATS	MILKS
	0	0
BREADS AND CEREALS	0	0	FRUITS AND VEGETABLES

NUCLEAR CAKE

I like to "nuke" a cake, meaning I put it in the microwave, step back, and hope for the best. I've had some incredible successes with this method. This amazingly simple recipe is one of them.

Serves 12

1 package Jiffy corn muffin mix   *sparkling water or diet*
1 package yellow cake mix   *lemon-lime soda*
4 egg whites, beaten

Mix together corn muffin mix and yellow cake mix; add egg whites and enough sparkling water or diet soda to moisten batter to cooking consistency. Pour into glass pan or casserole sprayed with nonstick cooking spray and microwave on low until cake has right consistency, approximately 7–10 minutes. While cake is still hot, cover with nonfat frozen yogurt (any flavor) or pudding, or cool slightly and serve with fresh fruit. Note: cooking time depends on microwave wattage.

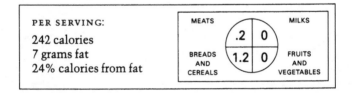

PER SERVING:
242 calories
7 grams fat
24% calories from fat

MEATS		MILKS
	.2	0
BREADS AND CEREALS	1.2	0 FRUITS AND VEGETABLES

*M*ix nonfat vanilla yogurt with nonfat whipped cream cheese and use as a sauce for fruit salads and as a topping for cakes.

CUTOUTS

These are messy to make, but children love to fix them. For Valentine's Day use cranberry-orange juice and heart-shaped cookie cutters.

Serves 16

1 loaf sliced whole-wheat bread　　*1 6-ounce can orange juice*
cinnamon　　　　　　　　　　　*concentrate, thawed (or*
　　　　　　　　　　　　　　　　　other frozen juice)

Heat oven to 250 degrees. Use cookie cutters to cut shapes from bread slices. Dip each cutout into juice concentrate and place on nonstick cookie sheet. Bake at 250 degrees until lightly toasted, about 20 minutes. Sprinkle with cinnamon. Serve warm.

PER CUTOUT:	MEATS		MILKS
87 calories		0 0	
1 gram fat	BREADS AND CEREALS	1.0 .4	FRUITS AND VEGETABLES
11% calories from fat			

HONEY CORN

Forget the Cracker Jack. Here's an almost fat-free flavored popcorn.

Serves 1

½ teaspoon honey　　　　　　*½ teaspoon water*
½ teaspoon lemon juice　　　　*2 cups air-popped popcorn*

Gently heat honey, lemon juice, and water until thin and warm. Pour over popcorn while tossing to mix thoroughly.

PER SERVING:	MEATS		MILKS
72 calories		0 0	
1 gram fat	BREADS AND CEREALS	2.0 0	FRUITS AND VEGETABLES
8% calories from fat			

25

Drinks

When I lecture, I ask my hosts to serve smoothies and low-fat muffins instead of the usual coffee and doughnuts. My audiences love the change. Here are a few of my favorite smoothies and other drinks.

RONDA'S SMOOTHIE

Serves 8

4 fresh peaches or 1 pint
  strawberries
2 ripe bananas

1 cup nonfat vanilla yogurt
1 cup nonfat milk

Cut fresh fruit into small pieces, put in blender, and blend until smooth. Add yogurt and milk and blend again. You can make the drink icier by blending fruit with 2 cups chopped ice.

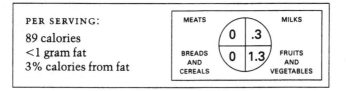

PER SERVING:
89 calories
<1 gram fat
3% calories from fat

MEATS · MILKS
0 | .3
BREADS AND CEREALS
0 | 1.3
FRUITS AND VEGETABLES

PEACH SMOOTHIE

Serves 2

1 cup nonfat milk
2 peaches, cubed

1 teaspoon honey
3 ice cubes, cracked

Combine all ingredients except ice in blender; blend until smooth. Add ice and whirl until frothy.

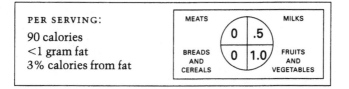

PER SERVING:
90 calories
<1 gram fat
3% calories from fat

MEATS · MILKS
0 | .5
BREADS AND CEREALS
0 | 1.0
FRUITS AND VEGETABLES

NECTARINE SMOOTHIE

Serves 3

2 nectarines, cut into slices   *3 ice cubes, cracked*
1 cup nonfat milk   *1 teaspoon vanilla extract*
¼ cup pineapple juice

Combine nectarines, milk, and pineapple juice in blender; whirl until smooth. Add ice and vanilla extract; whirl until smooth and frothy. Serve immediately.

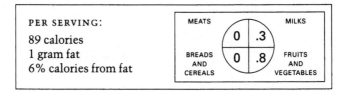

PER SERVING:
89 calories
1 gram fat
6% calories from fat

MEATS 0 .3 MILKS
BREADS AND CEREALS 0 .8 FRUITS AND VEGETABLES

FRUIT SMOOTHIE

Serves 6

2 cups nonfat frozen vanilla   *2 teaspoons lemon juice*
*   yogurt*   *2 cups crushed ice*
1½ cups sliced fresh fruit
*   (strawberries, peaches,*
*   raspberries)*

Combine all ingredients in blender or food processor and blend until smooth.

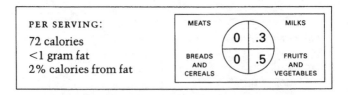

PER SERVING:
72 calories
<1 gram fat
2% calories from fat

MEATS 0 .3 MILKS
BREADS AND CEREALS 0 .5 FRUITS AND VEGETABLES

CANTALOUPE-NECTARINE SMOOTHIE

Serves 2

1 nectarine, cubed   *1 teaspoon honey*
1 cup diced cantaloupe   *3 ice cubes, cracked*
½ cup nonfat plain yogurt

Combine fruit in blender; whirl until smooth. Add yogurt, honey, and ice and blend well.

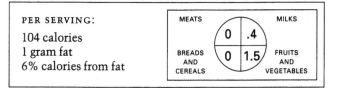

PER SERVING:	MEATS		MILKS
104 calories	0	.4	
1 gram fat	BREADS AND CEREALS	0	1.5	FRUITS AND VEGETABLES
6% calories from fat			

CANTALOUPE-BERRY SLUSH

Serves 4

½ cantaloupe   *1 cup nonfat strawberry frozen*
1 cup nonfat milk   *yogurt*

Prepare ahead: scoop cantaloupe into small round balls and freeze. In blender, combine frozen melon balls with milk and blend. Add yogurt a spoonful at a time, blending until slushy.

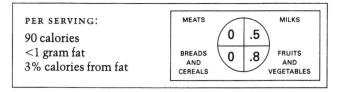

PER SERVING:	MEATS		MILKS
90 calories	0	.5	
<1 gram fat	BREADS AND CEREALS	0	.8	FRUITS AND VEGETABLES
3% calories from fat			

BANANA MILKSHAKE

Serves 1

When I was young, milkshakes were reserved for special occasions — or when I was ill. What a loss! These are good for you anytime!

*1 frozen banana, sliced into
    1-inch chunks
⅓ cup nonfat milk (adjust for
    desired consistency)*

*1 teaspoon sugar-free cocoa
    mix (or to taste)*

Blend banana chunks and milk in blender or food processor. Add cocoa mix to taste and process until smooth. Pour into glass and serve immediately.

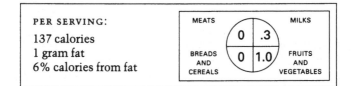

PER SERVING:
137 calories
1 gram fat
6% calories from fat

MEATS MILKS
0 .3
BREADS AND CEREALS 0 1.0 FRUITS AND VEGETABLES

ORANGE-BUTTERMILK SHAKE

Serves 2

*1 cup nonfat buttermilk
½ cup nonfat frozen vanilla
    yogurt*

*½ cup orange juice
2 tablespoons brown sugar*

Measure ingredients into blender; blend at high speed until smooth. Or beat with rotary beater.

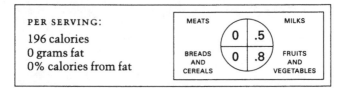

PER SERVING:
196 calories
0 grams fat
0% calories from fat

MEATS MILKS
0 .5
BREADS AND CEREALS 0 .8 FRUITS AND VEGETABLES

STRAWBERRY SHAKE

Serves 3

1 cup nonfat milk   *1 cup strawberries*
1 cup crushed ice   *1 cup nonfat strawberry yogurt*

Combine all ingredients in blender. Whirl until smooth and frothy.

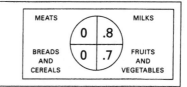

PER SERVING:	MEATS		MILKS
80 calories	0	.8	
<1 gram fat	BREADS AND CEREALS	0	.7	FRUITS AND VEGETABLES
4% calories from fat			

FRUIT FLURRY

Serves 8

3 cups fresh pineapple, chopped   *4 cups lemon-flavored*
1 tablespoon honey   *sparkling mineral water,*
1 cup seedless orange sections   *chilled*

Combine first 3 ingredients in blender or food processor; process until smooth. Pour into bowl or pan, cover, and freeze until almost firm. For each serving, scoop ½ cup of mixture into a glass; add ½ cup sparkling water. Stir well and serve immediately.

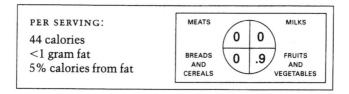

PER SERVING:	MEATS		MILKS
44 calories	0	0	
<1 gram fat	BREADS AND CEREALS	0	.9	FRUITS AND VEGETABLES
5% calories from fat			

PEACH FREEZE

You may substitute your favorite fruit for the peaches.

Serves 3

⅓ cup nonfat vanilla yogurt
¾ cup nonfat milk
1½ cups fresh peaches, sliced
1 tablespoon honey

crushed ice
peach slices or cherries
(optional)

In a blender or food processor, combine first 4 ingredients. Cover and blend until smooth and frothy. Serve immediately over crushed ice. Garnish with peach slice or cherry.

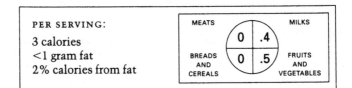

PER SERVING:

3 calories
<1 gram fat
2% calories from fat

MEATS	0	.4	MILKS
BREADS AND CEREALS	0	.5	FRUITS AND VEGETABLES

SANGRIA SLUSHER

The signature of sangria is the floating fruit. To make the traditional drink, mix half and half with your favorite inexpensive wine.

Serves 8

2 cups orange sections (about 6
oranges)
3½ cups fresh pineapple,
chopped
⅓ cup frozen lemonade
concentrate, thawed

2½ cups nonalcoholic Bacardi
mix, thawed (in supermarket
frozen-juice section)
1 cup club soda, chilled
8 fresh pineapple chunks

Put orange sections and pineapple in freezer bag and freeze until firm. In blender or food processor, blend frozen fruit until chunky. Add thawed lemonade concentrate and 1½ cups Bacardi mix; process until smooth. Pour into a large pitcher and add remaining 1 cup Bacardi mix and club soda. Stir well. Pour into 8 glasses: garnish each with a pineapple chunk. Serve immediately.

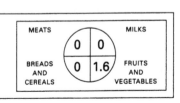

PER SERVING:	MEATS		MILKS
192 calories		0	0
<1 gram fat	BREADS AND CEREALS	0	1.6	FRUITS AND VEGETABLES
2% calories from fat			

HAPPY TIMES PUNCH

When I think of parties and punch bowls, this is the recipe that comes to mind.

Makes 6 quarts

2 6-ounce cans frozen
    lemonade concentrate
1 6-ounce can frozen orange
    juice concentrate
4 cups cold water

1 quart pineapple-
    orange-banana juice
2 pints pineapple sherbet
1 quart nonfat frozen vanilla
    yogurt

Combine frozen concentrates, water, and juice. Place sherbet and frozen yogurt in bottom of a punch bowl; break into small pieces with a spoon. Add juices and stir until sherbet and frozen yogurt are partially melted.

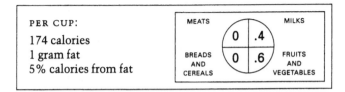

PER CUP:	MEATS		MILKS
174 calories		0	.4
1 gram fat	BREADS AND CEREALS	0	.6	FRUITS AND VEGETABLES
5% calories from fat			

EGGNOG

One glass of commercial eggnog has 19 grams of fat!

Serves 4

1½ cups nonfat milk
1½ teaspoons vanilla extract
⅓ cup nonfat dry milk
½ teaspoon nutmeg

2 tablespoons sugar
⅛ teaspoon salt
4 ice cubes

Blend all ingredients in blender at high speed until smooth.

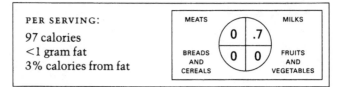

PER SERVING:
97 calories
<1 gram fat
3% calories from fat

MEATS		MILKS
	0	.7	
BREADS AND CEREALS	0	0	FRUITS AND VEGETABLES

Index

Covert Bailey has retired from public speaking. Clinics based on *The New Fit or Fat, Smart Exercise,* and *Smart Eating* principles are now directed by Ronda Gates. Like Covert, Ronda believes that to be successful, programs must be motivational, educational, and entertaining. She has developed products and workshops that support our message.

To learn more about living or teaching lifestyle behaviors or to schedule a lecture, contact Ronda at:

Ronda Gates
P.O. Box 974
Lake Oswego, OR 97034
Fax/Phone: 503-697-7572
Internet: rgates@teleport.com
Web Site: http://www.teleport.com/~rgates